Attitude
Affects Your Health

By

Margaret Mysiw

NOTICE OF COPYRIGHT

DEDICATION

With gratitude to the Creator I dedicate these writings to the memory of my loving and caring parents Clarence and Frances Zerbel, who by their example taught me the lessons of faith and love. My husband Steve Mysiw also was an inspiration in courage and patience. My family is the source of my strength to survive my trials.

Acknowledgements

I deeply appreciate the assistance given to me by my friends Annemarie and Joseph Quiles, who made an emergency retrieval from my word processor of my original work that otherwise would have been lost forever in my computer.

Secondly, to my friend Amy Mueller who helped convert my data to a format suitable for publishing including the technical layout and processing of the pictures found throughout this book.

Attitude Affects Your Health

By

Margaret Mysiw

Table of Contents

INTRODUCTION

This book has been written to inspire and encourage people to have HOPE. It is very important to develop a positive attitude. Your mind does affect your body to help the healing process. My intention of introducing my family first in the book is to show the importance of attitude and how it affected their life. This ultimately helped me with my pain and trauma. Most people (myself included) have peaks and valleys in their life. The peaks are the joyous times and the valleys are when illness and accidents happen. This is the time you use the memories of pleasant events to aid in your recovery. I call this the positive attitude of HOPE. My life has been filled with trials, but I found ways to enjoy my life and bring joy to other people. I have been fortunate enough to have good parents to influence my character. The impact of their inspiration would be tested many times throughout my life, due to the traumatic moments and events. My inner strength to cope would not have been possible without their early influences. They had a positive philosophy and practical wisdom, which looked at each day's pain or problem with the hope that tomorrow would be a better day.

These are the elements that would carry me through many unforeseen situations in the years ahead. My journey through life has had many ups and downs... I have had five cancer surgeries in the last twenty years and have dealt with diabetes the last ten. It is not my intention to fill this book with doom, but instead to inspire healthy strategies for survival and in a strange way—be a travel guide for your life. You will be surprised to read what I have done to enjoy life during this time. Skillful planning and constant saving allowed me to pay for my own enjoyment. My favorite saying is, "My life may not be exciting but it certainly is not dull". Hopefully you too will find my story enjoyable as I share my vacations, dancing, and the interesting people I have met on my life's journey. Worthy of note is the events usually followed trauma and surgeries.

My intent is to stress the attitude of HOPE for recovery. Have faith in God, trust your doctor's advice, and may my efforts be informative, inspiring and encouraging... Time to meet the family.

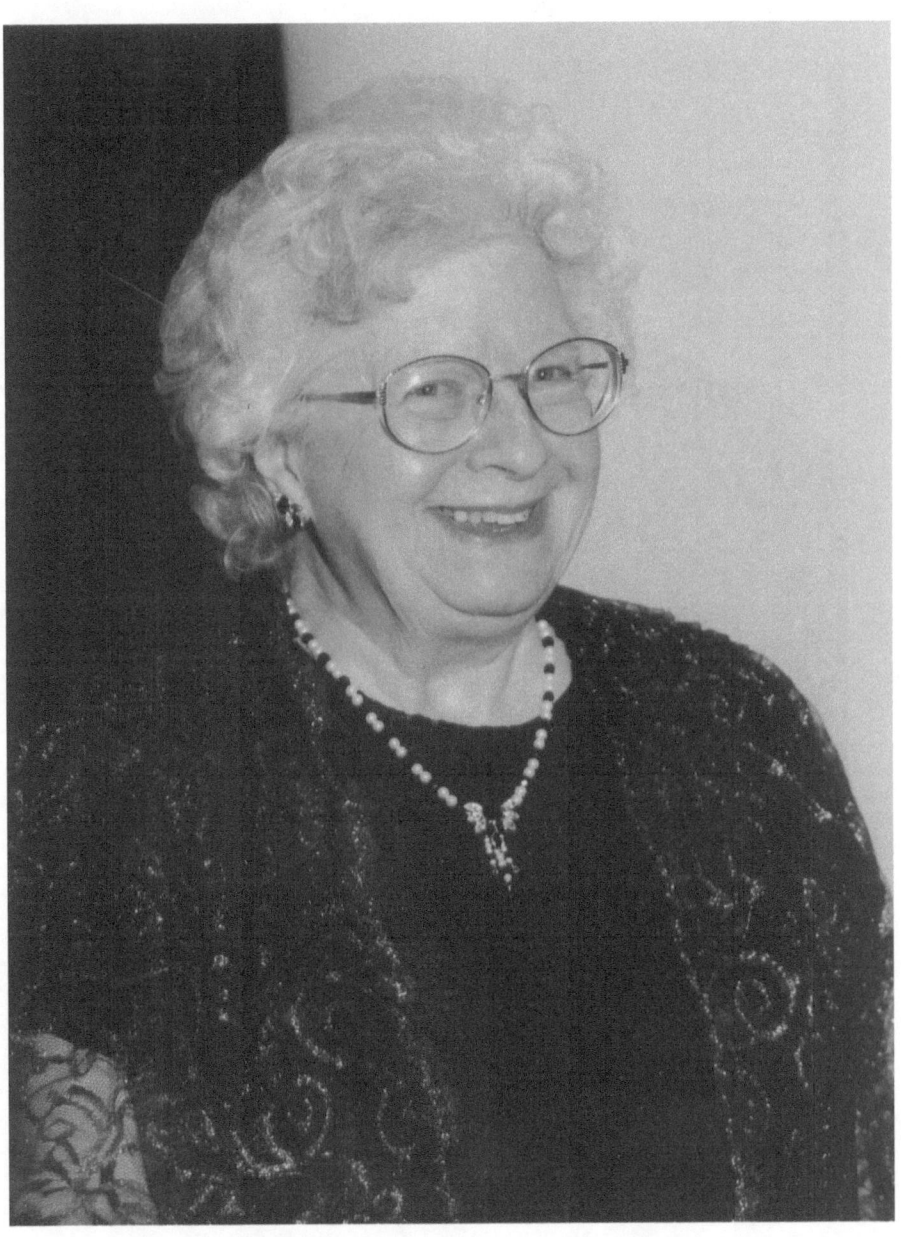

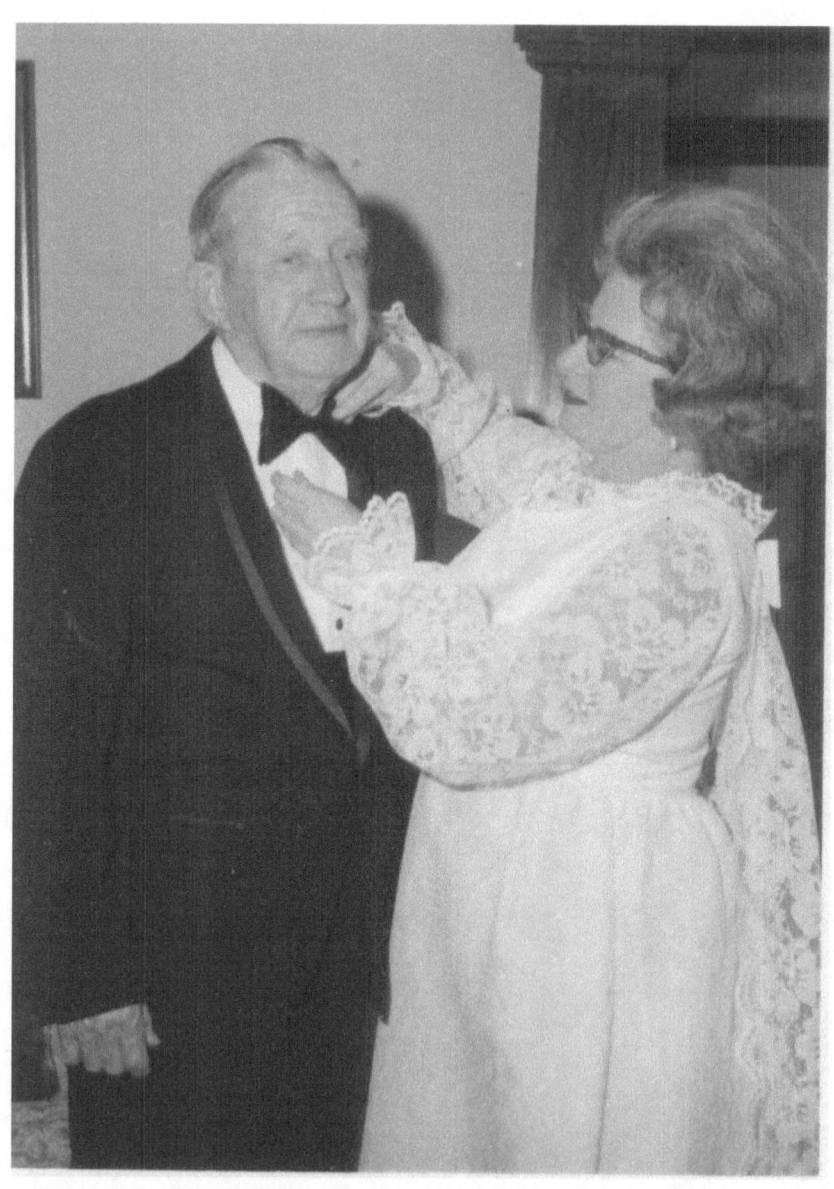

MY DAD

My dad's courage, perseverance and determination to survive did not just begin near the end of his life; rather, they were part of his entire life. It began about the age of 16 when both his parents died and he earned a meager salary to sustain himself. That determination to survive and provide led him to constant perseverance through the depression days of the early thirties. He walked 10 miles each day to work and many times walked the same distance home after working hard at his job. He was not a financial success but he was an overwhelming success as a husband and father. My dad was the greatest influence in my life. When I grew up all the lessons he taught by example were reflected in my decisions, my attitude and the development of my character.

Dad liked sports... especially baseball, and took me to parks near our home to watch the games. He took the time to explain what the players were doing and during the innings he promised to introduce me to the players. This was fun, and taught me to understand and really enjoy the game. As I grew older we listened to the New York Yankee's radio broadcasts along with other games. Baseball has become my favorite sport.

Music was our main enjoyment. Dad sang in the church choir and at home we would play music and sing at home together. He purchased a guitar for me, to inspire me to learn a new talent. He took an active part in my school activities. He set up chairs for school meetings, attended father and daughter breakfast meetings and was often found in the kitchen afterwards cleaning and drying dishes. On other occasions he would help serve the breakfast for this group. It was dad who helped me with my homework, which included catechism lessons. This is unique because my dad was raised Lutheran and allowed me to be raised Catholic. This mixed marriage had no problems with religion. Priest and ministers alike were always welcome in our home and both were guests at dinner for social events.

Dad was also active in his church. He seldom missed Sunday services. He had a nice tenor voice and said he liked to use it to praise God. At one time he was a member of the church choir. When the ladies at church needed help in setting up chairs and tables for their activities my dad would volunteer to help. After dinner or luncheon functions you would find him in the kitchen washing or drying dishes.

Dad was well liked by the church people for his kindness and willingness to be helpful. For his 85th birthday the members gave him a surprise birthday party. A large cake was delicious and attractively decorated. Dad got numerous cards and gifts, had a sing along, and then they packed some of the cake so he could take it home to Mom and me. I think what Dad enjoyed most was that his friends remembered him and the evening closed with a brief sing-a-long.

Birthdays were events that were always celebrated at home in some manner. We would invite a few friends for a party and for most of the time buy a decorated cake. One year I ordered a cake for Dad's party with a music record on top. When I went to cut the cake… you guessed it—the bakery had mounted the decoration on cardboard, and as I cut the cake the knife hit the cardboard in such a way that the decoration flew across the room. We all had a good laugh and enjoyed a delicious cake. My embarrassment enhanced the fun evening of playing records and singing songs. Dad truly loved music, so we spent many summer evenings at the Washington Park Pavilion when it featured the orchestras and barbershop quartets in their programs called "Music Under the Stars" (sound familiar?)

Dad also enjoyed what he would call 'mini trips'. These were one, two or three day tour guided trips. These trips included Wisconsin Dells, the Minneapolis Aqua Follies, Johnson Wax Company, the Holland Michigan Tulip Festival, Mississippi Boat tour, the Lady of the Snow Shrine in Belleville, IL, and the Buckingham Fountain in Chicago, IL, just to name a few. All these trips were interesting to him and dad added to the pleasure of others with his cheerfulness and friendliness to others. Dad had a special gift—almost an energy that exuded from him—that made people he met happy to be with him.

In the year 1948 my parents had their first chance to take a lengthy tour when they celebrated their silver wedding anniversary. It was similar to the one I had taken the year before to Washington, D.C., New York City and Niagara Falls. It was my gift to them, and they enjoyed the entire trip. The boat tours were a new experience for them. We took a boat ride on the Potomac River in Washington, D.C., and a ship to the Statue of Liberty in New York harbor. They were especially amazed at the magnificent beauty of Niagara Falls. They originally saw the falls during the day, and then we returned at night when colorful floodlights made the scene more dramatic and beautiful. This was absolutely breathtaking.

In the years that followed we took more small trips, including a trip in 1954 to the Holland Michigan Tulip Festival. We saw the tulip farms, the dancers that wore wooden clogs in the parades, and the street sweeping. There was a souvenir store where you could even have your own clogs made to order. We enjoyed our mini trips, but life was about to change.

In 1960 our faith was given a real test. Dad's doctor gave us the shocking news that Dad needed major surgery for colon cancer. We were completely in shock, and cried our hearts out. The day of surgery quickly arrived. Mom and I assured Dad we would be there to help him and care for him, no matter what. This was a long painful day for all of us.

After the operation and a lengthy recovery period, my Dad resumed his performance of charitable works for his family, friends and the church. During his recovery the members encouraged him by sending him cards, some visits. He lived with a colostomy for 18 years in such a manner that people were not aware of the many times he had discomfort or pain. He would gladly go shopping not only for my mother but for the neighbors as well. He was happy to be able to go to church again and volunteer at church functions. After dinner or luncheon functions you would find him in the kitchen washing or drying the dishes.

My fun loving father was always there to listen to my problems because my mother was ill a great deal of the time. Dad never forced his opinions on me, but rather provided guidance toward the solution of the problems. I remember when I was a teenager I met a divorced man for whom I developed a serious relationship. I really wanted to marry him but it was a big decision. The Catholic Church strongly opposed such marriages, which meant I would have to leave the church if I married this man. I told my dad of my dilemma and as usual he made a simple statement to guide me toward a decision. I was a very devout Catholic and active in the Catholic Church. Dad said, "Honey, ask yourself this question. Will I be truly happy and at peace if I marry Eddie and give up my religion?" I decided to sever this friendship.

In the early 1960's the Catholic Church made sweeping changes. I found some of the changes hard to accept and once again I confided in my dad on a very important issue, namely, of joining his Lutheran Church and changing my religion. He told me to think the matter over carefully but to keep in mind the importance of having faith in a Supreme Being no matter what church I might join. These are only two examples of major decisions or reasons why my dad and I had such a strong relationship. Dad encouraged me when I needed encouragement and consoled me when I felt sad. . My joys were increased and problems resolved by sharing my thoughts with him.

Most of my youth was spent as a single person caring for my parents sharing joys and trials with them. Then in 1972 I made a decision to marry. A proud father walked hand in hand with his daughter down the aisle to present "his little girl" to someone else. Even though I was a mature woman, my dad always referred to me as "his little girl". There was a noticeable sadness but also a look of unselfish happiness for his daughter. He appeared satisfied that Steve was a good man my husband was accepted as a son rather than a son-in-law. Family events from then on would include my husband, Dad and Steve became pals, sharing and enjoying similar interests.

In 1973, my parents celebrated their Golden Wedding Anniversary. Neither of my parents was feeling good that year so we did not want to do anything too strenuous so we decided on an elegant place called the "Columns" which would serve a delightful dinner while we enjoyed listening to a very good orchestra.

In 1974 we had a special surprise for his 80th birthday. My husband purchased tickets to take dad to listen to music played by Jack Morgan and the Orchestra that was playing at George Devine's Ballroom. We enjoyed an exquisite dinner and an evening of dancing at the ballroom. We went up to the stage during the intermission and told Jack Morgan that it was dad's 80th birthday and he asked what some of his favorite songs were. The remainder of the evening, the Morgan Orchestra played several of these tunes. We spent a delightful evening dancing and singing until the last song was played. We left the ballroom with long lasting memories.

In the summer of 1974 we took a conducted tour to Michigan to visit the Kellogg Cereal Company this trip also included going to the Ford Museum and Greenfield Village. The Henry Ford Museum had attractions of old memorabilia that was too numerous to remember. Dad and Steve liked to reminisce about old cars, trains, the potbelly coal stoves, musical instruments and they talked as we walked to other exhibits. Airplanes attracted me .A duplicate plane of the "The Spirit of St. Louis" that Charles Lindbergh made his solo flight across the Atlantic in 1927 was on display. The original "Spirit of St. Louis "is housed in the Smithsonian National Air and Space Museum in Washington, D.C.

On May 21, 1927 Charles A. Lindbergh completed the first solo non-stop transatlantic flight in history, flying his Ryan NYP "Spirit of St. Louis" plane. He left Roosevelt Field on Long Island, New York and arrived at Paris, France in 33 hours 30 minutes. This was an outstanding event. The second plane on exhibit was that of Admiral Byrd, a Naval Officer who flew an expedition to the Arctic (North Pole) in 1928. We were on a time schedule. We left to go to Greenfield Village another site of outstanding interest. The home of Steven Foster displayed his music. The homes of inventors Thomas Edison, Alex Bell and many others for whom we can be grateful for our current conveniences, showed even more.

In July 1978, Steve and I decided to take Dad on a one-day tour of Chicago. It was only one of the few times that my mother did not care to go with us. We had a wonderful time especially the boat cruise. We mixed with many of the people and near the end of the cruise we joined in with a group who were singing songs. This was the last tour for my dad.

In August 1978 the third critical surgery was performed as the result of a rupture in the colostomy area. During the surgery he went into a comatose stage that lasted almost three months. He was not expected to live and the life supports were removed after a week in the Intensive Care Unit. He was moved to a room near the nursing station for close observation. I visited Dad every day and after a month there appeared to be no change in his condition. Then I had an idea that I thought might help. Someone had told me that hearing was the last of our senses to go dormant, so I taped some records that dad enjoyed. I played his favorite music each time I went to see him. After playing the music a few weeks I noticed my dad turned his head to the side where I was standing. When I moved to the opposite side of the bed and played the music then he turned to that side. I reported this information to the nurses. The next day a television set was playing when I visited my dad but the nurses reported the television playing had no effect on him. I continued to play the tape recorder and one evening dad opened his eyes! Progress was made in his condition.   The nurses and the doctors called him: THE MIRACLE MAN". No one expected him to live, much less come out of the coma. As time passed, more progress seemed to be made. The nurses began to have him sit in a wheel chair in the corridor so he could see people. At the end of three months, arrangements were made to put dad in a nursing home to get therapy.

At the nursing home he had very strenuous exercises. The therapy eventually made it possible for dad to use a walker. He progressed enough to bring him home for one day during the 1978 Christmas holidays. The following month of therapy was completed so my dad was released from the nursing home. When he came home he walked with the use of the walker. But soon dad exchanged that equipment for a cane. With the use of a cane he went for short walks to visit neighbors or go to the grocery store with me. Near the end of the year he was walking in the house without a cane. Dad was easily satisfied and the smallest kindness was rewarded with a warm smile. However, he seemed a little sad at Christ time 1979 and he remarked, "I think this is my last Christmas," I asked if he felt alright and he said, "Yes I am alright" and added quickly "let's play some music."

After the holidays it became necessary to place dad in a nursing home again because my mother and husband were not well at this time. I felt I could not give adequate care to all three of them. At the nursing home he did some dusting and small chores for the nurses. He found it difficult not to keep busy. Three months later he had a cold and that developed into pneumonia. He was sent to a hospital on April 25th and the next day in the early morning we received an emergency call. We were told the next 48 hours would determine the outcome. In the meantime the nurse noticed my mother was having some problems. Upon hearing of her existing heart conditions, the hospital staff temporarily placed mom in another room to give her oxygen and monitor her condition .I spent several hours going from her room to dad's room to check on the condition of each parent.

There was little I could do except to bear the grief and anxiety. Close to the noon hour, when my mother was more stable, the hospital released her and told me to take her and my husband home. I went back to the hospital again alone because Steve was not up to par. Near supper hour I returned home to see how my family was feeling and we decided to eat a light meal at a restaurant on the way to the hospital. While we were eating we heard the 6:00 church bells chime and I felt a strange sensation that something was happening. "I said I can't eat any more-we are going to the hospital now". As we walked into the hospital a nurse met us and she said that at 6:00 my dad died. I stared in disbelief and the tears could not come out. I told the nurse I could not cry and that I felt a severe pain on the inside, which I could not explain. She said the tears will come later and then you will feel some relief. I watched my dad and the quiet way he accepted his pain and suffering through the 20 years of surviving Colon Cancer surgery and his daily struggles to walk after coming out of the coma. April 26th, 1980, my dear dad died of pneumonia. This was a great loss to me, my mother, my husband and all whose lives he had enriched by his pleasant manner, thoughtfulness and numerous good deeds. This indeed was a painful experience to have this brave cheerful person leave me.

MY HUSBAND - STEVE

Steve met me at the place of my employment a short time after serving in the military. He had just had an honorable discharge November 1945 from the U.S. Army Air Force after 4 ½ years of service. During that period he sustained a permanent eye injury and also developed allergies and asthma. This was the beginning of a life of suffering. VA performed nose surgery to aid his breathing. The federal building underwent repairs and walls were demolished causing dust and asbestos to be constantly inhaled by Steve in his working surroundings. He became extremely ill and developed Blastomycosis. The treatment for this lung disease took months to cure and caused a collapsed lung. The extensive medication left him with a new ailment— Diabetes. He was in and out of the hospital repeatedly for chronic asthma attacks and diabetes but both became worse as the body was treated with various medications. He still continued working and trying to enjoy his life as much as possible. During these many years his co-workers, including me, would visit him in the hospital. My mother met Steve one Sunday morning when she and I were walking home from church. She was impressed by the courteous manner of the young man who had tipped his hat as he passed by. She said, in a very definite manner: "There is a very nice young man. Where did you meet him?" I told her that occasionally we would double date and go to baseball games, we worked in the same building on the same floor, and that he had recently moved into our neighborhood. She further stated: that compared to all the other men I had invited to the house, she could not understand why I had never invited Steve. On Thanksgiving Day, we did invite Steve to our house for dinner. He impressed both my parents.

Since we were neighbors, Steve and I frequently rode the same bus to work in addition to seeing each other at work. We did date occasionally going to various sport events, shows, festivals and office parties throughout the years. However, Steve never pursued a steady courtship

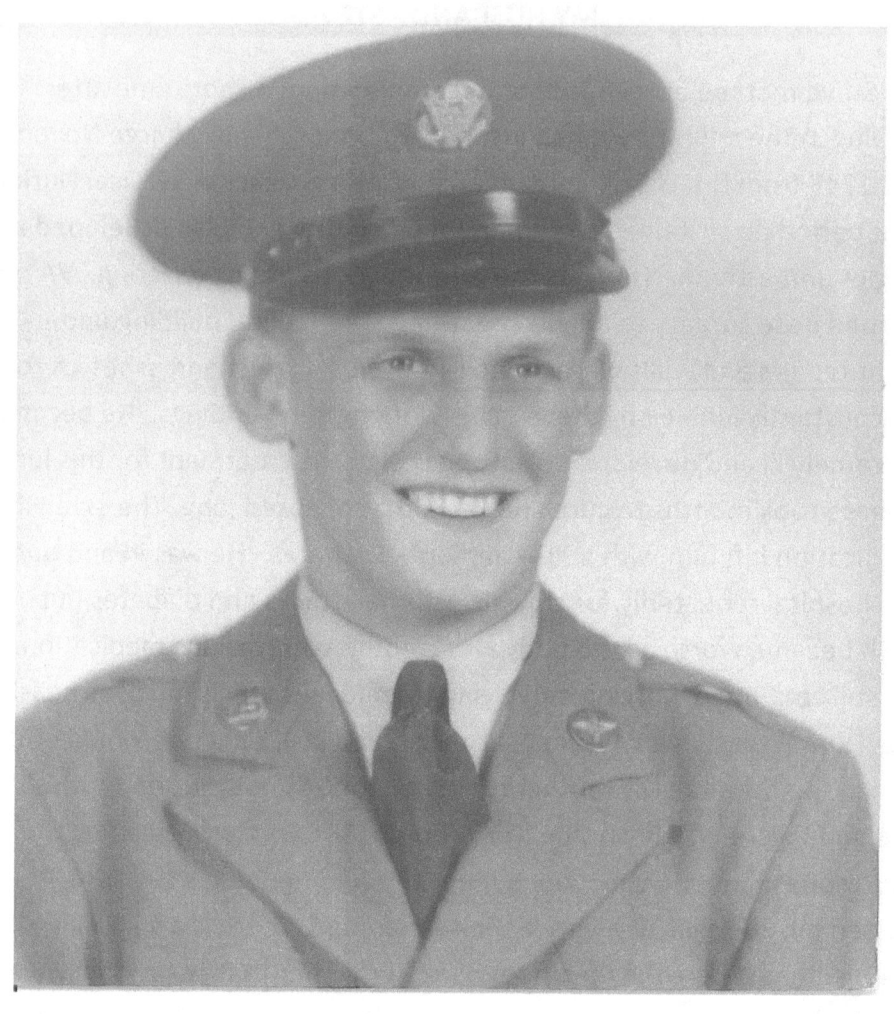

Cpl. Steve Mysiw

Dates of service

June 4, 1941 - November 16, 1945

due to his health. He was a very thoughtful, concerned person and exhibited these traits to all who knew him at work and he certainly showed these traits to me on numerous occasions. Everyone we worked with felt that we would be an ideal couple. Our co-workers would frequently urge each of us to take the initiative toward a serious relationship. It would be many years before marriage would become a reality. In the meantime I dated many other men and one more frequently who would pick me up after working hours. Steve showed some concern and wanted to date me again. A short time later, just prior to the Christmas Holidays, we went to Southridge Shopping Center with me believing it was to be a window-shopping spree. However, at each jewelry store Steve would stop and look at the display. I told him I was not interested in any more pins or necklaces. He said, "No, I want you to look at engagement ring and wedding rings." I was surprised but found out that this was his way of asking me to marry him. We were engaged and set our wedding date for October 7, 1972.

Preparations for the wedding did not flow smoothly. In fact, Steve was hospitalized in February 1972 with chronic asthma and a diabetic reaction from medication. Some of our wedding plans were made and others were put on hold until Steve showed improvement. About the same time, my dad had to have surgery due to a rupture in his colon. After the recovery of both, we proceeded with our wedding plans as scheduled. I was well aware that our marriage would have its periods of turmoil.

Our big day came and we had an abundance of happiness to start our marriage. Our friends and co-workers were delighted. We had approximately 100 guests and about 75% of those present were co-workers. We hired a number of our co-workers to provide our services. One man made a beautiful centerpiece for our main table. The three-piece band was composed of one of Steve's co-workers along with his son and friend. The photographer was a co-worker who was an experi-

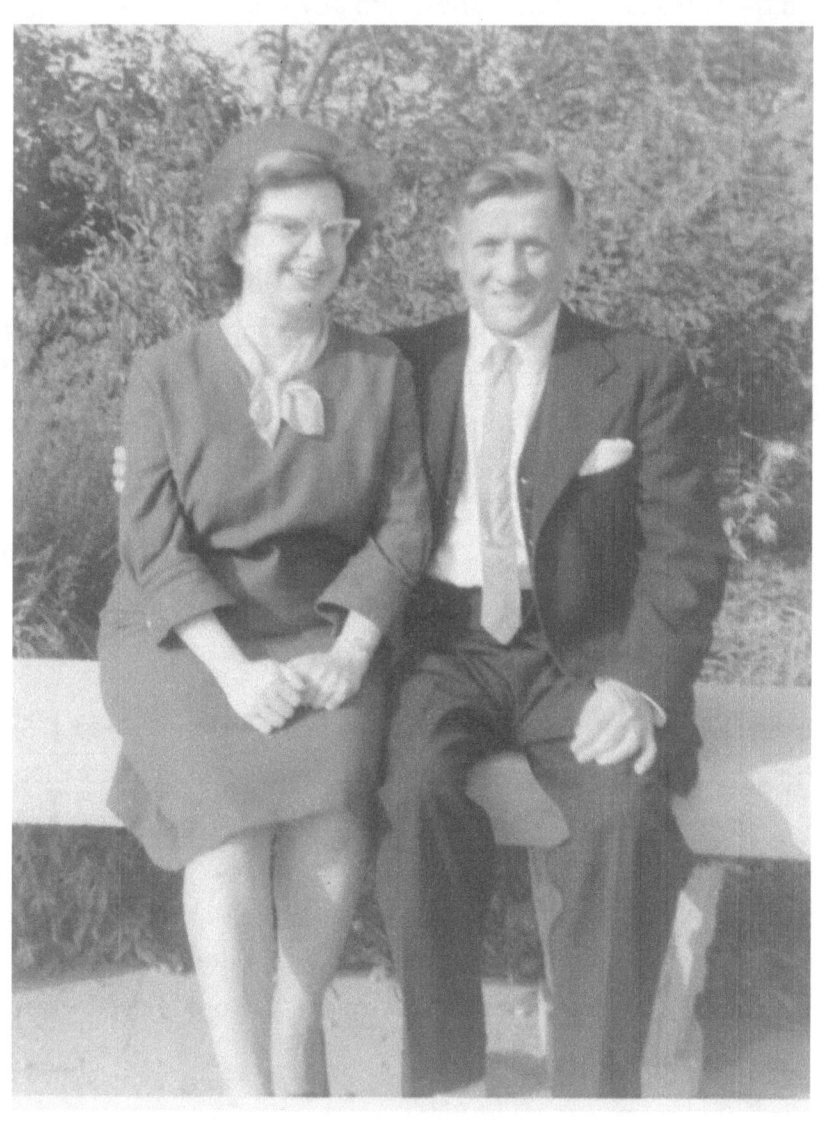

I met Steve Mysiw at work

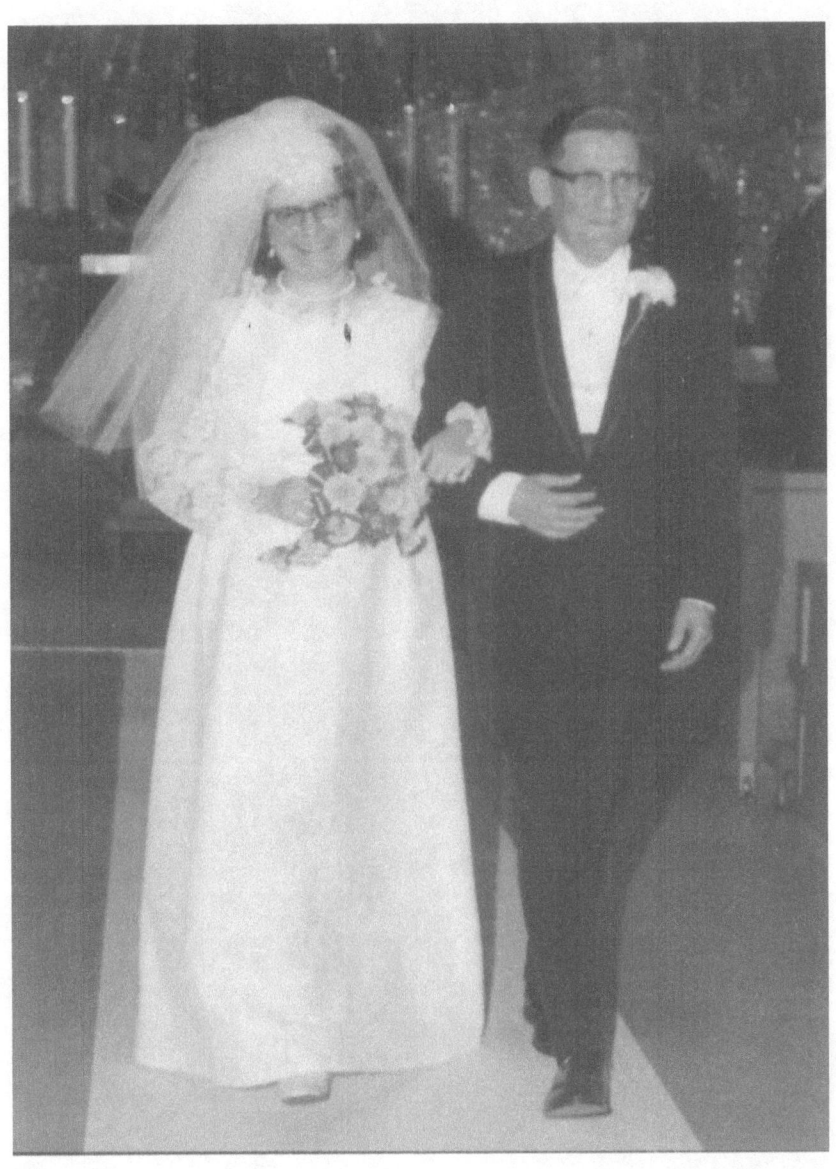

Margaret & Steve Mysiw

Wedding day October 7, 1972

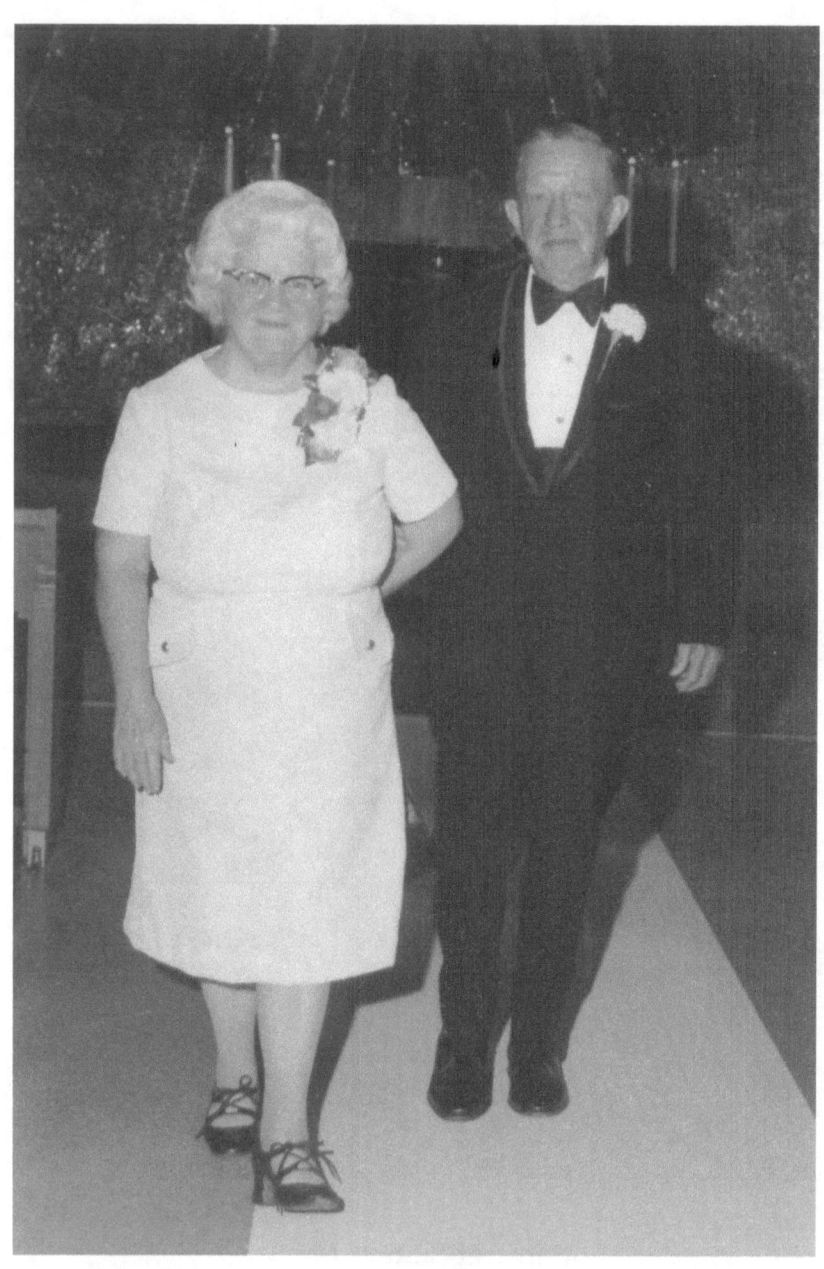

Dad & Mom

Clarence & Frances Zerbel

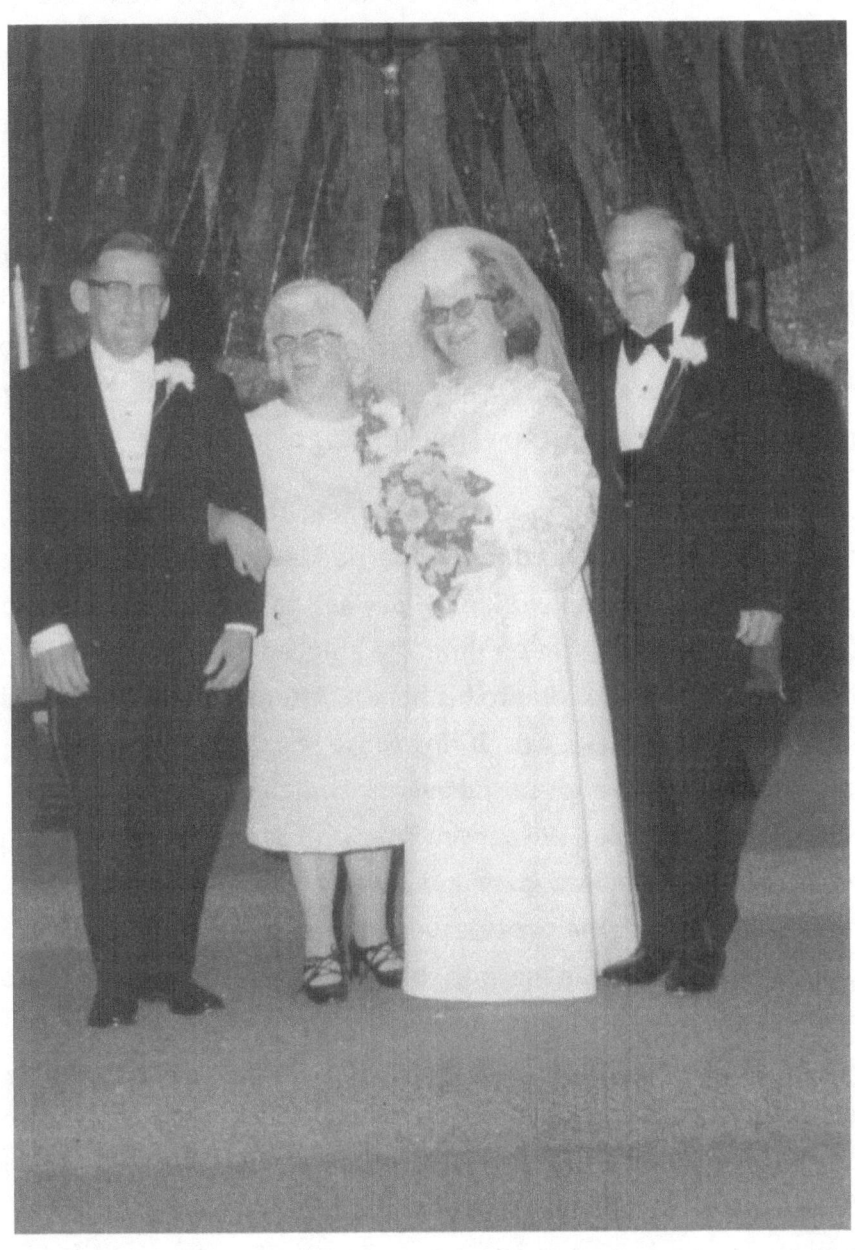

enced U.S. Navy photographer. Steve's best man was a friend and former neighbor. Steve's brother Frank and another fellow were also a part
of the wedding party. My three bridesmaids wore light blue formals.
One was Steve's niece Debbie, one was the daughter of the best man
and the third was one of my best friends, named Honor.

The church service and music were nice. Although we were an older
couple, we had all the excitement, joys, dining and dancing which are
normal for any young couple. The following day we flew to Florida for
our honeymoon. We visited Disney World, Kennedy Space Center and
took a number of bus tours to various places of interest.

Happy with the memories of our wedding day and trip to Florida, we
optimistically looked forward to our married life. Our life for the most
part was routine, going to work each day and taking care of household
duties. When we had vacation time, we enjoyed taking small trips
rather than lengthy ones due to his health. After we married his health
seemed to improve and it was during those few years that we enjoyed
most of our vacations and special events. One of our favorite places was
the Shrine at Dickeyville, Wisconsin. The Grottos and fences around the
gardens contained colored glass and jewelry from all over the world
imbedded in cement. The Grottos were impressive and the flowers were
beautiful. The Shrine was the work of a priest who did most of this creative beauty over a period of many years before he died. My parents,
Steve and I took this trip to Dickeyville and stayed at a nearby motel for
three nights. During the daytime we took additional trips to nearby
sights of interest. One such trip was to Prairie du Chien to visit a Victo-
rian-style mansion. The mansion was built in 1870 on land that was
owned by Colonel Dousman and his son Louis. This place is called "Villa
Louis" named after Colonel Dousman's son. The Dousman family was
the earliest, richest fur traders in Wisconsin. Their lifestyle was that of
bountiful living and entertaining other prominent people of their day.
The tour included the fine works of art, attractive china, silverware,

glasses, furniture and exquisite clothing of the 19th century. The mansion was both educational and beautiful. Villa Louis was a very interesting place to visit but we had a frightening experience on the way back to Dickeyville. We were driving at the normal speed when suddenly the car did not seem to move. Steve had a good deal of knowledge about tornadoes because of his early training in the Civilian Conservation Corps camps. As he looked at the sky he consoled me by telling me constantly, we were not moving because we were on the edge of the tornado and we were not in any real danger. I kept my foot firmly on the gas pedal and at last we were able to move slowly around the mountain. We later found out about the tornado damage and we were extremely happy that we had not been at a more precarious spot. That evening, the electric power went off at the motel in Dickeyville, but we recalled the nice events of the day and we were all grateful for our safety.

Another family trip was to the Wisconsin Dells. The boat trip to the Upper and Lower Dells were very impressive with the huge colorful rocks and crevices and unbelievable formations. There is a boat at the Dells that has the capability to be used on land as well as water and the vehicle is called a 'Duck'. Steve said it reminded him of his army days when riding in a jeep was so bumpy that milk could be turned into a milk shake on the rocky terrain. This ride was better because from a rocky land ride you splashed into clear smooth refreshing water. Mom and Dad accompanied us on most of our trips. Steve liked my parents very much. His choice was to call or refer to them as Mom and Dad right from the beginning of our marriage. My parents in return were very good to Steve and treated him like a son. So it was no problem to have my parents with us on trips. Steve and I did take a few trips by ourselves. We went to Chicago in April of 1977 to view the King Tut Exhibit. We went on a tour of the Johnson Wax Company, Sara Lee Bakeries, and the West Bend Aluminum Company.

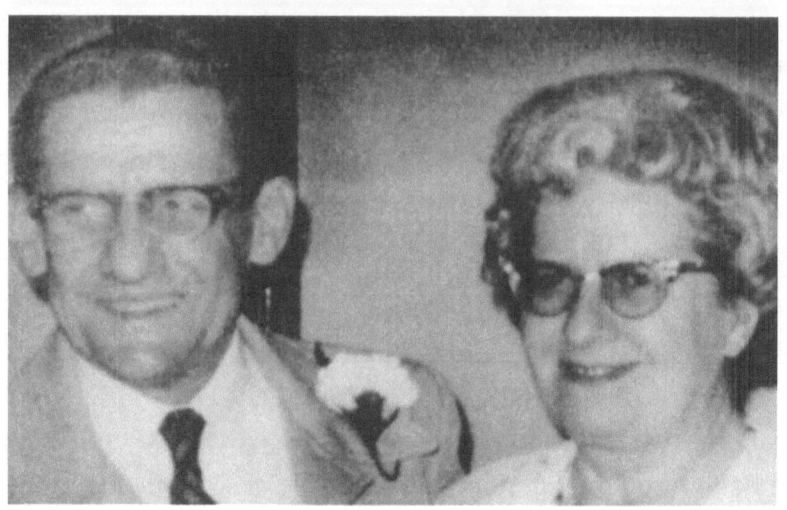

October 1977 we celebrated our 5th Anniversary

In October of 1977, we decided to celebrate our 5th Wedding Anniversary in a special Manner. Since we were older when we were married, I approached the parish priest and asked if we could have an Anniversary Mass to publicly repeat our marriage Vows. I told the priest that for every year of our marriage, we figured it was equivalent to five years for a young couple. He said the idea was unusual but was happy to go along with the idea. I am glad that we did this, even if the idea seemed odd to some people who did not understand. To us we were celebrating our 25th Anniversary because we believed we would not have a chance for that special event mostly due to health reasons. That evening, we had several friends share a nice dinner with us.

In 1978 & 79 we took a few more short trips. We went on a Cherry Blossom Time Tour to Sturgeon Bay and attended a delicious Fish Boil cookout. One of Steve's favorite tours was to the Shrine of our Lady of the Snows at Belleville, Illinois. He enjoyed this peaceful atmosphere. He purchased a few religious articles to add to his memorabilia.

This seems an appropriate time to point out that all of the illness and pain really helped us to appreciate the good days of joy and happiness that we sandwiched in between by means of our vacations, birthday parties, picnics as well as wedding and retirement parties of our former co-workers.

November 1979 was the onset of Steve's stroke. He went to the Veteran's Hospital for his flu shots. He had a reaction from the shots, even before he left the hospital. His face swelled, his eyes watered, he felt dizzy and his arm swelled. I was at work and he called for me to take him home because he was sick. I was frightened when I saw his condition and called the V.A. hospital. I was told to call back the next morning. That evening he had ringing in his ears that continued on and off. The Veterans Hospital personnel denied that these conditions were caused by the flu shots. We went to Steve's family doctor and his doctor made light of this condition saying that when you get older a lot of aging conditions develop. My husband was only 59 years old at that time. I made an appointment with my doctor but by this time all efforts were too late. In 1980 the disaster struck as my husband had a major stroke. I was informed that the ringing in the ears, the dizzy spells and the blurred vision were small strokes known as TIA's which usually precede a major stroke. I do believe that had the proper diagnosis been made of all those symptoms the major stroke would have been avoided.

On April 26th 1980 my dad died of pneumonia. Steve made phone calls for me that evening. The next day Steve was an ashen gray, he could not swallow even water. I drove him to St. Francis hospital which was only one-half block away. The personnel admitted him first as an outpatient but within an hour, admitted him as an inpatient. I told Steve I would be back as soon as I made dad's funeral arrangements. When I returned to the hospital the doctor told me that my husband had suffered a stroke, and his chances of survival were very poor. Steve's stroke paralyzed his right side. He tossed violently from side to side. Because he knew he was in serious condition. He used his left hand to reach out to me, and tried to say something and in desperation he cried. I knew he could understand me so I told him I would get the best possible care to help him. In the days and weeks that followed, I made daily trips to the hospital to visit him and check on the progress. The nurses advised me that he refused to eat after his intravenous feedings were discontinued and that they were lucky to get him to take orange juice for breakfast. I decided I needed to be there to encourage him during his noon and evening meals. I would feed him a little at a time of whatever was on his tray: Jell-O, pudding, soup or ice cream in small portions. I talked to him throughout his meals, urging him to eat just a little more. Then one morning, he suffered from a bleeding ulcer and was returned to the Intensive Care Unit and this time it didn't look like my husband would survive. However, by this time I think, Steve had gained a little more desire to live. I spent a good deal of time telling him that therapy could help him to become mobile again. So even in his critical condition, he seemed determined to get better. During the two months at St. Francis Hospital, his means of communicating was by pointing to pictures on a card, which did not always explain his needs.

At such times, it was very frustrating for Steve and very difficult for me to figure out. When he began to show improvement, the hospital advised me that my husband needed rehabilitation therapy; On June 1st St Francis Hospital staff transferred Steve to Sacred Heart Rehabilitation Hospital.

STRUGGLES FOR MOBILITY

At Sacred Heart Rehabilitation Hospital, Steve underwent strenuous exercise and training in an effort to become mobile and to learn to talk again. He received physical, occupational and speech therapy. He learned how to eat with his left hand, to do limited grooming and dressing activity and to formulate some words. In addition to this he learned to maneuver his wheelchair. I visited nearly every day to encourage him and to check on his progress. In the meantime, the personnel taught me how to transfer Steve from the bed to the chair. The therapist instructed me how to transfer him from the wheelchair into my car. I was advised that he would not make further progress and therefore the choice was mine to either send him to a nursing home or take him home. My choice was to bring him home, which meant a great deal of preparation was necessary. A short time before his release two therapists came to the home. They suggested fixtures for the bathroom, and recommended the door way be widened. A ramp was necessary because I was not strong enough to manage the wheelchair up and down steps .I received instructions on how the ramp was to be built and the care to be given him. The time approached for Steve to come home and it became a very emotional time for him. The tears rolled down his cheeks as he tried to tell me that if I took him home, I would have to dress him. He felt he would be too much of a burden and was not satisfied that he could not do more. I assured him, it would work out alright. I took him home on the first day of September. He was very depressed because he felt he would not improve any more. He had a strong desire to walk and the first night home, he fell out of bed because he had dreamed he could walk again. Panic struck me. How would I get him back to bed? We used the technique for transferring after Steve worked with me to get into the upright position. The next day I ordered a hospital bed with side rails which proved to be very helpful. As time went on, Steve lost interest in sports, wouldn't even watch television; didn't want the shades up during the day; didn't care to eat. I became very concerned and decided to seek additional therapy elsewhere. I made arrangements to have a visiting nurse come to our home twice a week to teach Steve some exercises. The nurse taught him to partially dress himself. This task was difficult and I was proud of his efforts to take on this new struggle for mobility. In the meantime, I began using my left hand to eat and did other things with one hand to understand the efforts Steve was making to adjust to his handicaps. I did these experiments while he would take an afternoon rest in bed. I didn't want him to develop a complex of feeling he was a burden. Even sitting in his wheelchair to try to ride over the carpet gave me a sense of how he was struggling.

In October, the Curative Rehabilitation Center consented to take him; as long as he would show some progress, they would continue therapy. Steve began a series of exhausting therapy. He was fitted with a leg brace which weighed five pounds. With the aid of a therapist he learned to walk the parallel bars. In speech therapy he learned to form words. I attended all his sessions so that I could continue the therapy at home between visits. His speech improved as I used a tape recorder to let him listen to his words and practice improving sound. His daily struggle to recover rewarded him with showing improvement. Therapy continued until July, a total of ten months. At that time, we were told he would not improve much more. In the meantime, Steve had finalized his work career and retired. His former co-workers planned a nice dinner party and gave him thoughtful cards and gifts of all kinds. Many of his friends remarked about how well he was able to talk. By that time, Steve was able to talk very well. Actually to the point where he could easily answer the telephone for me when I was busy, or when his friends would call to speak to him. His walking continued to be difficult because he could not balance due to the extent of his stroke, and the complications of asthma, which made breathing difficult. I contacted the veterans' hospital to see if additional therapy was available there. The veterans' hospital did provide another three months of exercise therapy and occupational therapy so that Steve learned how to do some arts and crafts even though he had the use of only one hand. He made several gifts for me, including a very nice trivet composed of small pieces of tile placed in such a manner as to form an attractive design. Another was pair of copper wall plaques. One had the image of the head of a horse and the other had a ship with sails. One craft was made by winding string around nails that were placed in Styrofoam. All these things are deeply treasured. He also learned to write with his left hand. Steve was encouraged, and we both accepted this as the end of outside therapy help.

Time out for a caretaker too. This brings up another worthy point. Many nursing homes now have Respite Care during the day to allow a spouse free time. This care is available for people with strokes or those who have other chronic ailments. These care centers also provide various types of recreation during the day as well as a meal or two, depending on the number of hours spent at the facility. This Center was an aid to me when my mother returned home after her surgery and I needed time to care for her. So Steve spent a short time at the center before I could be available for both of them. I occasionally was a volunteer at some events when needed. People who have spare time could be contributing valuable time to a worthy cause.

TIME OUT FOR PLEASURE

After two years of working together on Steve's efforts to become mobile and to try to talk, we decided that in 1982 we would try to enjoy our lives. Steve had always wanted to go to visit Holland, Michigan during the tulip time festival and he now felt this would not be possible. However I told him not to give up because I intended to find a way to take this long dreamed of trip. In the meantime I wanted him to have some form of recreation. We enjoyed the Greater Milwaukee Stroke Club which gave us a chance to meet other people with disabilities. The meetings were once a month and were very interesting. They provided some enjoyable entertainment such as sing-a-longs, speakers and Christmas parties. In the summer we had picnics at parks. I also found out about a Daycare Center at a nursing home. This nursing home had just started this program and my husband was the first to enroll in the center on March 17th, 1982. He liked this activity; in fact, they had a St. Patrick Day party the first day he attended. He was excited about being taken to a local bar and drinking green beer. Steve went to the day center about three times a week for a while. The group took trips to movies, the zoo, some of the parks, to the Summerfest grounds and various other places. I was asked to join the group once in a while. I also planned little side trips to the parks or movies. Occasionally we went to see the Circus, Holiday Folk Fair, parades and an indoor skating show called the Ice Capades. I did not give up on the Holland Michigan Tulip Time Festival. I made numerous inquiries. Finally I made arrangements with a van company that transports handicapped people in an effort to obtain a van and driver. The effort was successful. The trip to Holland Michigan was made possible through the co-operation, kindness and generosity of the president of the company Mr. Len Lovdahl. He made available to us his own private van and his own driver to take my mother, Steve and me to the Tulip Time Festival.

On April 24th, 1982, I contacted the Tulip Time Housing Authority; I informed them that my husband was in a wheelchair so that would be considered in making plans for proper housing accommodations. Confirmation was received with a program and map. This made it possible for me to organize and plan each day's activity before arriving in Holland Michigan. We saw many interesting events. There was a concert with a large chorus of men and women in formal attire. Another event was a dramatization of various aspects of Holland History and a colored slide presentation on the making of the wooden shoes. We watched a large parade from an excellent viewing area. The van driver, Mr. Bob Wilson, had a great skill at moving the wheelchair in and out of the crowds with little confusion. We watched people scrub the streets before the stores opened. Even little children in wooden shoes and costumes used small brooms to participate in this Holland tradition. Later that day we drove to a tulip farm where there were acres of many tulip varieties featuring a rainbow of colors and combinations of colors. An impressive sight to behold! Steve was able to see his dream come true. The entire trip went very smoothly and we had a wonderful time.

In the month of May 1983 my mother became sick due to a gall bladder problem which later required surgery. I arranged to have Steve in the nursing home at the location of the Day Care Center. During the two months as a resident, he was on the Welcome Committee for any new in house resident. He knew many of the regular residents from greeting them when he came for the day for activities. I took care of mom when she came home from the hospital and managed to visit Steve nearly every day. After two months I brought Steve home from the nursing home.   In September we were invited to a wedding and in October we went to another wedding. We had a nice time at both of these events and the same month one of Steve's co-workers retired. So we attended this retirement party as well as many others. We went to movies, the circus when it came to our city and the yearly Summerfest event and most of the ethnic festivals.

ALL WAS NOT PLEASURE

As you read about the recreation and trips, you might find it hard to believe that this warm, cheerful man was enduring simultaneously a wide variety of suffering and painful treatments. He was in and out of hospitals frequently during 1984 and 1985 due to a variety of his ailments. He had allergy, asthma attacks and his urinary infections were very painful. His fluctuating blood sugar also caused problems. He was on a rigorous diet and various amounts of insulin combinations prescribed by the doctor. I followed the instructions religiously, but diabetes was difficult to control. He almost lost his eye-sight due to an infection. The treatment for the eye infection was cured and his eye-sight saved. How did he accept this almost continuous life of suffering? Like a true soldier. He endured all the old and new treatment in a very courageous manner. Many doctors and nurses at the VA commented that they admired his patience, attitude and endurance.

Steve had a good sense of humor. Once in a while if the phone rang, he would take a message for me to return the call. My dad passed away in 1980, if the caller would ask for my dad Steve would find out what the caller wanted. If the call was someone selling something Steve would reply, "Dad is not home." If the person asked when he would be available Steve replied, "I don't know he is out bowling with his friends." When mom and I heard that response we all had a laugh. This is one example of Steve's humor. We played tricks on him too. One Christmas we put a boiled egg in a container resembling a piece of coal and wrapped in a fancy Christmas box. They were just simple things to put a little laughter in our lives.

Steve was a religious man, he liked to go to church when the weather was nice or when he felt well enough to go. The priest from the parish came with Holy Communion on the first Friday of each month. Steve would kid with the priest, talk sports and politics jokingly. He would tell the priest about some of the people at the nursing home and remark that he was lucky to have the comforts of home. The recreation planned for my family brought them some pleasure and relief from pain and it helped me as the caregiver. It was a source of consolation for me after their deaths, during my adjustments to their loss, because it left me with some pleasant memories.

For a family such as mine with the amount of trauma, sickness and serious ailments it seems almost unreal that we worked in as much recreation and pleasure into our lives as we did. It was not easy to do because it took planning, cooperation, patience and a cheerful positive attitude on the part of each of us. Mother, Dad and Steve were never a burden. I consider the care of each of them as a labor of love.

Our house: A Home of Love.

Love: can overcome obstacles.

Happiness: can be found in accepting each day....as a challenge instead of a burden.

Pleasure: can be mixed with pain.

Help from God: can make all things possible.

In 1986 Steve was hospitalized four times and his health conditions became worse. His body began to reject all the medications and even the type of insulin had to be changed. Recreation became very limited. He spent most of his time working jigsaw puzzles when the weather was inclement. It was remarkable how he could put the large puzzles together with the use of only one hand. Many puzzles were over 1500-2000 pieces and he could finish most of them in less than a month. Steve was easily satisfied and was content to sit on the porch in the summer time and watch the children next door playing. Sometimes he played his radio to listen to the ballgame or some nice music. His warm friendly smile was still present even though it became evident that he losing the zest to live. One day in November 1986, while sitting on the porch Steve was told the neighbor next door had died. When he heard the news he said, "Why did Carl die? Why couldn't it have been me? After all Carl had two good legs to walk around on." That summer I spent a great deal of time working in the yard and this bothered Steve. He did not like to see me working in the garden, while all he could do was watch. When I was aware of his feelings I discontinued this activity.

Many of the times that he was in and out of the hospital may not have been necessary had he received the proper care from the doctors.

At this time I wish to state that I feel most doctors do care and try to help their patients. Unfortunately there are doctors who are thoughtless and look at the patients as another job to make money. They have little or no concern for the process of healing or treating the patients with respect. I think my husband was victimized too often by this type of doctor.

I feel very sad that my husband did not have the good professional doctors that I was fortunate to have in the years of my serious illness and surgeries. Perhaps I should have been more insistent in his care but I tried to honor his choice.

On January 31, 1987, Steve and I attended the wedding of Rick and Patricia Lopez, who were longtime friends. This beautiful wedding was to be the last big social event for my husband and me.

His last day of recreation was on March 19th, 1987. Steve and I went to Pabst Mansion which is the historic home of the founder of the Pabst brewery. It is a lovely home and interesting facts were revealed about each room. The home reflects the beauty and the architect of the past years very well. Our tour of this home was very interesting and enjoyable.

After a delightful day my husband had a restful night sleep. Little did I realize as I watched him sleeping pleasantly that night that in less than a month he would be taken from me.

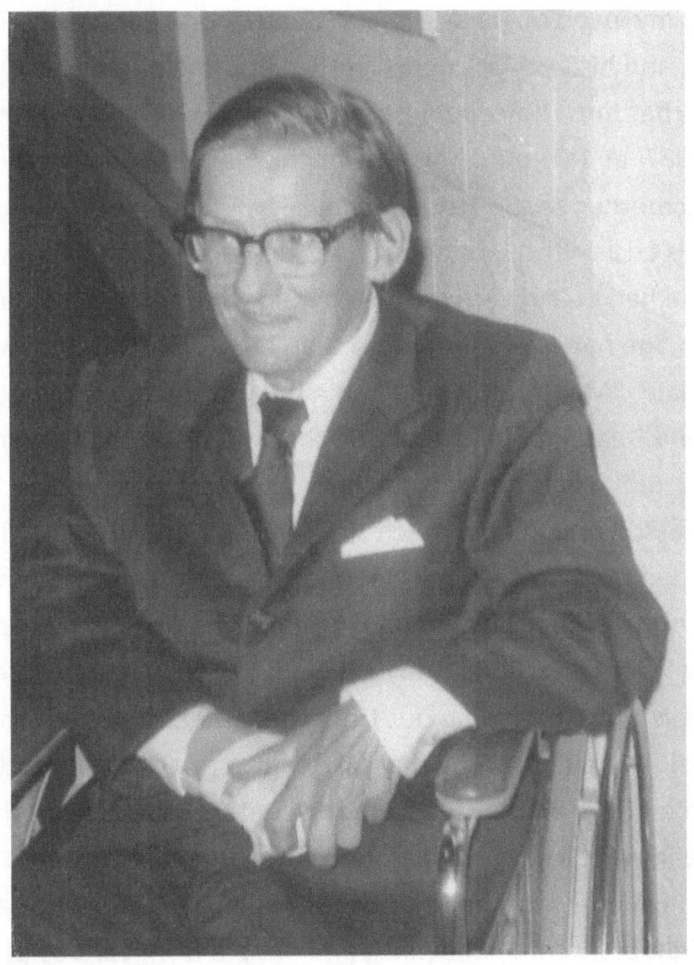

STEVE'S FINAL DAYS

Steve was in the hospital only two days before he had a stroke on the opposite side of the first stroke. He lapsed into a coma that lasted five days. This was the beginning of the Easter weekend   I felt I was living the Passion of Christ. I sat at the bedside in the Intensive Care Unit knowing that part of my life would be leaving me in a few hours. I was aware that my loved one was close to death. I prayed silently. Then I kissed him, and his eyes opened slightly. I told the nurse and she smiled and said, "That must have been some kiss." Steve died Wednesday, April 15, 1987, at 1:05 a.m. This was my husband's Good Friday. I hugged my mother as she stood by me. Her warm embrace helped me through this crisis. I thought about how lucky I was to still have my mother. She had been there for me so much during the final days of Steve's life. She had loved him more than I realized. This was evident when she said, "Margaret, would you mind putting the words, 'Beloved Husband and Dear Son' on the ribbon that will be on the flowers over the casket? Steve was more like my son than just a son-in-law." This really impressed me on how much she cared for my husband. It is not hard to understand how we had so much pleasure and co-operation in our family during those last pain filled years. The regular vigil and the military vigil were on Good Friday evening. There were many people at STEVE'S vigils   who took time out from the busy Easter weekend to bid him farewell. People from the day care center (many in wheelchairs) as well as some of the employees from the center. Friends from the stroke club (some in wheelchairs) some of his Army buddies, former colleagues with whom we both worked, friends we had made before he had the stroke, neighbors, some politicians, and people from various professions.

He was well liked by people from all walks of life. Steve had full military honors bestowed by members of the American Legion, Veterans of Foreign Wars and the Disabled Veterans. On Holy Saturday, The full rites of Christian burial could not be celebrated because of Holy week. Prayers and blessings were meant to comfort us in the interim of the Memorial Mass. The ushers' society with whom he served at church formed an honor guard in the morning at church. The priest accompanied us to the cemetery for the final prayers at the cemetery chapel. It was so consoling to see that so many people cared. The wide range of Steve's involvement was evident by the presence of professional and non-professional people who were at the vigils. HE HAD LIVED A FULL LIFE in spite of all his sufferings, and even confinement to a wheelchair did not keep him from touching the lives of all those who came to know, love, and respect him.

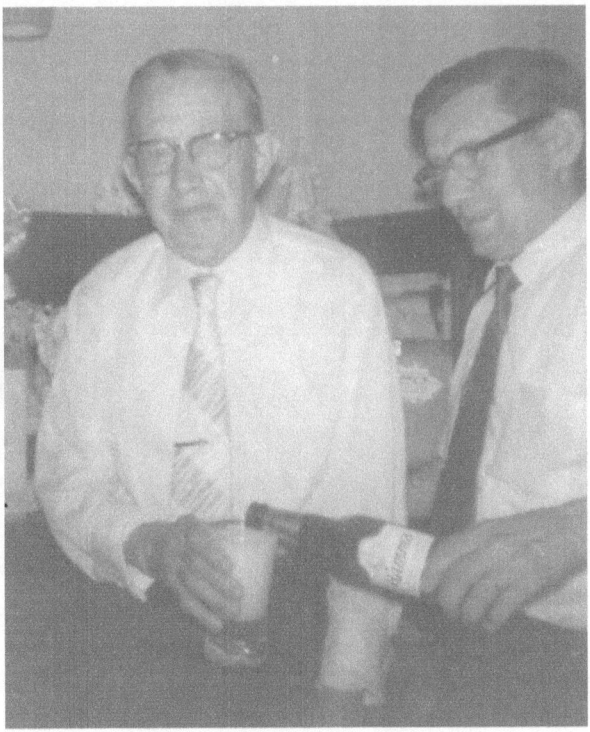

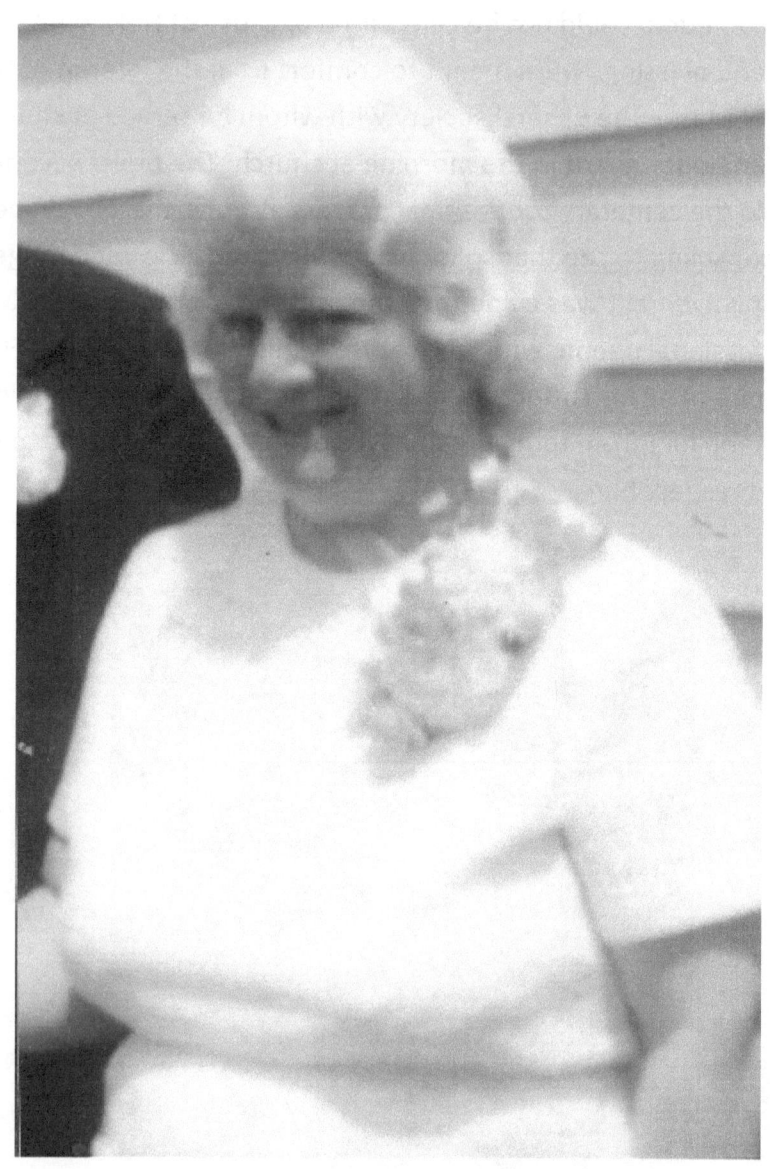

MY MOTHER

You have been introduced to my dad and my husband. Now it is time to meet my mother. When my mom was about five years old her family moved from Waukesha to a home located at 38th and Greenfield Avenue in Milwaukee, Wisconsin. That area at that time was surrounded by dense forest called "Koepsell's Woods" and the Indians in the area were family friends. Mom told me that her father sold goods to the Indians and would cut their hair for them. The Indians liked him and the family. My mother was the youngest child of the large family. The Chief was especially fond of my mother and wanted to give her an Indian pony. She was greatly disappointed when her dad would not let her accept the pony. Mother related the story of how Gypsies sometimes would kidnap children and keep them. The Indians were very protective of her family.

As the years passed Mom witnessed the growth of neighborhoods she mentioned that neighbors in those years were more caring than people are today. She told me how one neighbor lady saved her life when she was a growing child by providing her mother with containers of goat's milk. At that time mom was troubled with a stomach disorder and the colic. The goat's milk diet helped cure her. This is one example of neighborliness of times gone past.

My mother almost died when I was born but she had a very strong faith. I was born at home (a breech baby) and during the entire birth process my mom clenched her rosary in her hand. From what my dad told me the imprint of the beads remained for quite a while. The doctor had said that he was not sure he could save her and only her faith would bring her through. My mother's stamina and strong faith went together. She prayed as if everything depended on God, then worked and disciplined herself as if everything depended on her own efforts. She learned discipline in her childhood from her father who was strong on discipline and equally strong in faith.

One of my fondest memories of early childhood was a hot summer day, when I was about four or five years old. It was too hot to go out to play, so my mom spread a quilt on the front room floor and we pretended we were on the beach. We had cookies and soda and we played a game of jacks and a small ball, plus a few other games. Mother had a good way of playing games with children. She would make kites for all the children that played with me. She would give us articles so we could pretend we were operating a grocery store, and she would help us make a tent to play in and to shield us from the sun on very hot days. She played games with children of all ages. She had creative suggestions for them on hot days, cold days or windy days when outdoor play was not practical. Neighborhood children looked forward to the sweet treats in the form of homemade cookies or cake or a cool drink of juice on a hot day. When any of us sustained a bruise, mom was quick to give first aid treatment. Besides her love of children she liked her hobbies of growing plants and caring for birds. There is an expression known as having a green thumb and she had a special knack of growing a wide variety of plants, which was her hobby until her death. She had a number of well-trained canaries. She would be able to let them out of their cages and get them back again with very little difficulty. Mom as well as dad would feed the sparrows and other birds in winter and in summer. Some birds would actually peck at the windows to be fed. Mom would fix broken legs of birds and when they were well again, they would fly away. She took abandoned baby birds and fed them with an eye dropper until they could eat by themselves. Her life was a life of love, a deep faith and love of God. Then her love went down the line to people, children, plants and birds.

When I was about eight years old my mother began having real health problems. Mom began teaching me how to cook, and at times when confined to bed would give me detailed instructions on the preparation of food from her bedside. When Dad came home, he would finish anything which I had not completed. Her life had several periods of hospitalizations due to coronary heart disease and various types of surgery. Mom had a major heart attack about 30 years prior to her death and was not expected to live at that time. A short time after recovering from the heart attack Mom had a light stroke, from which she also recovered. During the good times between illnesses she enjoyed our mini trips which we had as a family, as well as a good baseball game and picnics in the park.

The year 1980 was filled with hardship. That is the year my dad died. My mom assisted me in making the funeral arrangements. She seemed strong in handling her own grief at the loss of her husband while trying to console me in the crisis of my husband's stroke which happened the day after my dad died, and I was informed not to delay the funeral but instead to prepare for the death of my husband. Even in poor health, mom continued to perform tasks which amazed me. She helped me a great deal to adjust our home life when it became neces-sary to move furniture and belongings into her home after Steve sur-vived this stroke. Merging two households under any circumstance is hard enough but under my conditions, the word could be chaotic if it were not for the splendid manner in which my mother helped me. She was a TOWER OF STRENGTH! I was a little surprised at the manner in which my mother accepted Dad's death and the apparent ease of ad-justment she made in her life. Within a few weeks she was humming or singing while I was torn with grief. She told me, "Dad suffered enough, now he is at peace, so I am at peace too." She had a strong faith which seemed to give her additional strength.

My mother gave me a great deal of help and comfort in the days and years that followed dad's death. She felt sad that I was angry with God for permitting all the tragedy to befall me. My faith already had been weakened earlier because of all the changes in the Catholic Church. Now I was more confused and believed God was punishing me unnecessarily. I decided to separate myself from the Catholic Church.

Mom started her crusade of prayers for the next seven years so that I would return to the Faith. She repeatedly would say "God is good; don't blame God". She would pray long hours into the night; I believe she was praying in her sleep for me. She was happy near the end of her life because her prayers were answered when I returned to the church.

When my mother was 83 years old she had her gall bladder surgery. This was a serious operation, especially for a woman of her age and heart condition. The morning of her surgery I was with her. She held my hand and said; "Don't worry about me. I have faith in God and I trust this surgeon I would be very surprised if I didn't survive the operation." My mother then started to laugh for she realized what she had just said. How could she be surprised if she didn't survive the operation? It would mean she had died. Just about this time the nurse came in to give her an injection and the attendants were about ready to put her on the gurney to take her to the operating room. The attendants remarked they had never taken a patient to surgery laughing. After the operation, her surgeon, Dr. Jack Herrington, asked about the story that made mother laugh. He told me Mom was a remarkable person and added that she came through the surgery very well. Both of my parents had a good sense of humor and a love of life.

In 1985, my mother had a cataract removed from each of her eyes. She was so happy about seeing things clearer that she wanted to take a scenic trip. My husband consented to go to a Respite Care Center for a week. Then Mom and I took a tour to Canada which included Algonquin Province Park and a long train ride around the mountains. In April 1987, my husband died. Once again, Mom was my TOWER OF STRENGTH. She reminded me of the good things which I had done for Steve and told me that his death was not in my hands. He suffered a great deal, and Steve had said, "Mama I don't think anyone can help me now. "Mother said that he spoke those words while I was grocery shopping the same day that I rushed him to the hospital when his breathing appeared extremely serious. She thought that if I knew how he felt, it would help me adjust to his death.

That summer we had the wheelchair ramp dismantled and remodeled the porch according to Mom's specifications. She only enjoyed this porch a couple of times before her death. In October my mother had two heart attacks. Sweetest Day was celebrated on October 17, 1987 while my mother was in the Intensive Care Unit. I bought her a bunch of pink baby carnations for this special day. On the card I wrote "To the Sweetest of the Sweet." The flowers and card made her feel happy. That was the last time I would bring her flowers on Mother's Day, May 8, 1988, and as I reflect on her smile that day, I also remember words she often spoke. I would ask her what could I buy for her on Mother's Day and she would reply, "Honey, I have Mother's Day. Every day of the year because of the love you show me." It is true that I did not wait for special occasions because anytime I saw something she might like I bought it for her. This is a comfort to me now. She did get well enough to come home for a short time before she died. When she arrived home she was surprised by a newly acquired rocking chair. I had ordered some cushions from a catalog, but the cushions for the chair arrived the day of my mother's funeral. The arrival of the cushions gave me a feeling of panic. Someone said, "You must console yourself with the things you did provide for her."

On Saturday morning, November 7th, the day Mother died, I came home from Mass and gave her Holy Communion, which is something I had done several times in the previous weeks. She received the Communion Host before being taken to the hospital in the ambulance. That afternoon Mom said, "Margaret, if I survive this heart attack it will be a miracle, after all I am 87 years old." She was alert to the end; she seemed at peace that I was near her. That evening at 6:25 my mother died. Mom knew how to make her final exit from life graciously and peacefully. I hope I have learned from her how to do the same. My mom's death was the saddest day of my life. She was the last member of my family. I felt I no longer had dreams to dream. I was overwhelmed with strong emotions of sadness, anger, guilt and loneliness. Family support and love had helped me before through trauma and sorrow. I had to deal with this grief all alone. In the following chapters I will reveal the manner used to survive my grief and trauma.

PENNIES GROW DOLLARS

This chapter may seem strange to be inserted before going on with the rest of my life's story. I believe it is necessary because I began my life in the days of the Great Depression. It also explains how my lessons of saving and thrift made it possible for some of the joy and trips to help my parents prior to their death. During the Depression, Dad walked 10 miles each way to and from work for very low wages. There were times when dad found it necessary to charge groceries but he paid the bill in a timely manner. Clothes and other necessary household items had to be charged at times to be paid over a certain length of time. As usual dad paid on time. He had very little life insurance but he cashed one in to pay his bills. He tried to avoid paying interest because he said, "interest is lost money". My mother shopped for healthy food and still tried to buy the cheapest and the best. I think sacrifice was the name of the game. As a child I saved my pennies to give my dad bus fare so in bad weather at least he could ride one way. My mother did not work outside the home because dad wanted her to take care of me. When I grew older I too got a job. When I graduated from grade school I won a two year Fellowship to a high school, which paid for half the tuition. During the summer any money I earned I applied to next year's tuition. The same was true for my final year of high school.

After high school graduation I obtained a full time job. Each time I received a raise that portion was put in a savings account. As the years passed by the government issued certificates of deposit (known as CDs) which had higher interest payouts. So, I purchased them from my savings account. Much later in my life I bought Annuity Insurance which would later be a supplement to any pension I may receive.

My husband was somewhat similar in this way. When it was time to assign our pensions, we each decided to take reduced pensions so that it would help the surviving spouse.

Dad always said there was a difference between need and want. If you need something, you spend the money. If you want something, you save for it. Thus, I saved for pleasure and was able to take those nice trips, and bring some joy to my family and husband. These savings also helped me to survive my surgeries and traumas.

In the current economy, the amount of credit and charging for things has hurt this generation, who may find it difficult if not impossible to do as I have with my life. However, maybe some part of my life's story may help your situation.

TIME TO MEET THE AUTHOR

As I have unfolded this story, you have shared in the joys and trials of my family. Perhaps you would now like to meet me. In April 1947 my parents faced the possibility that their only child might die from a Ruptured Appendix. The incident happened on a Sunday afternoon while visiting friends. I was rushed to the hospital and surgery took place early evening. After the operation the family doctor who was an excellent surgeon said the poison had traveled through my system and he told my parents after the operation I had about a 50-50 chance of survival. I was in my early 20's but I looked so young that I was put in the children's ward, until I regained consciousness and was safe to be transferred to an adult ward. In the meantime, I was given penicillin injections every 3 hours around the clock for two weeks. Thanks to Dr. Schodron's skill and treatment. This good doctor saved my life.

After a few months of recovery, I decided to plan a vacation with a co-worker. We decided on a tour to Washington, D.C., New York City and Niagara Falls. The first place on our tour was our nation's capital. We visited the Capitol, the Library of Congress, part of the White House, the Washington Monument, the Lincoln and Jefferson Monuments, the Immaculate Conception Church and other churches of historic interest These are only a few of the many places of interest we enjoyed during our brief stay, and they still remain in my memory. We boarded our bus in Washington, D C. for our next destination which was New York.

This trip had its share of excitement too. The events were laughable after the trip but a little nerve wracking in the experience. One bus had a flat tire while traveling through the mountains. Another bus we were on had a seat which slid forward every time we hit a bump in the road, the window did not stay closed and in general it was in poor condition. We were stranded in Scranton, Pennsylvania because of motor trouble. Most of the passengers found lodging for the night, or had Scranton as their destination. We asked the driver when the next bus was due in town. We told him of our concern about our tour connection, and the driver suggested that we flag down the bus which was due about two o'clock in the morning. He made no promise that we would have success. Late in the afternoon his bus was towed away.

Picture, if you will, two young women outside a dimly lighted bus depot waiting for a bus which normally would just pass through town at the suggested hour in the morning and not scheduled to stop for passengers. We waited patiently and then we saw the bus arrive. We both waved our arms frantically to stop the bus. The driver saw us; opened the door and told us the bus was filled to capacity. He told us there would be another bus at six in the morning and we should wait for that bus. We briefly stated our dilemma about the disabled bus and our willingness to stand in the aisle. We explained the urgency of making another bus connection so we could continue our vacation tour. He repeated, "No seats available!" and was about to close the door. We offered to sit on our suitcases in the aisle. By this time, the passengers were awake and glared at us for disrupting their sleep. It was a very rough ride but we were content to be on our way. We arrived in New York to make our next connection to the Big Apple. In New York we enjoyed many delightful experiences, including a performance by the Rockettes (the precision dancers) at Rockefeller Center, and a boat trip to the Statue of Liberty. Other highlights were a tour of the Empire State building and attending other musical shows. There was a great deal to see and so little time to include all the events and places.

Finally, it was time to move on to the last place on our agenda, the Niagara Falls. We saw the grandeur of the falls during the day and the spectacular beauty at night with all the colored lights magnifying their wonderment. At last, when we came to the end of our vacation, we found that we had taken all of our problems in stride and the trip ended up being more of an adventure than anything.

In my youthful years, in addition to vacation trips I was actively engaged in church activities... Examples: such as helping with the parish newsletter to servicemen, which was printed once a month, teaching Sunday School, and doing charitable works which included visiting homebound people and inpatients in nursing homes. The parish organist established a girl's chorus which I enjoyed. We sang at various events including entertaining at the Veterans Hospital. Each year the parishioners looked forward to our formal concert. This was a colorful event with all the girls wearing pastel formals, beautiful flowers and a background displaying the theme chosen for the concert. After several years the chorus group was discontinued.

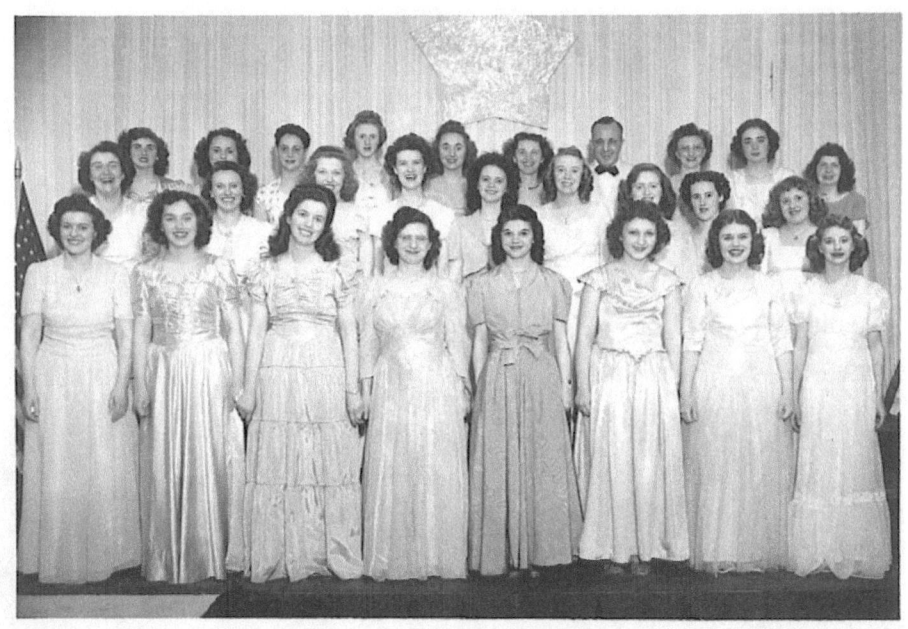

My other form of recreation was dancing. I took dancing lessons twice a week and frequently dated fellows from the classes. I was dating some of these men when I met Steve who worked for the same employer. Steve dated me on and off for fifteen years prior to our marriage Oct 7th 1972. He later told me he delayed the thought of marriage because of his health problems. It is regrettable that the marriage was delayed because the years we were married were very happy but illness was almost a daily companion. Frequent visits to doctors for Steve and occasionally for me were common.

MATURE YEARS

I had not told Steve that most of my life I lived with a painful intestinal condition. I saw many doctors and no one could diagnose my problem. In fact, some even implied that it was my imagination. Then one doctor discovered that my colon was not normal. He drew a diagram on a card and told me to carry it with me at all times. If I collapsed at any time no one would know the reason or how to help me. I would have to learn to live with the condition. My dad went to Dr. John Hurley for one of his problems, and told him about my condition. Dad made an appointment for me with Dr. Hurley's office at St Mary's Hospital. When Doctor Hurley saw the diagram he assured me that my condition although very rare was still correctible. This surgery would require the reversal of the large colon and removal of the extra footage of small intestine. I was aware that this surgery was critical. My odds would probably be 50-50 but no other doctor would take any action to help me. In 1976, my parents agreed with me that I should have this surgery. I had full confidence that this surgery would be successful. I was willing to entrust my life into the capable and skillful hands of Dr. Hurley, who was well known to be an outstanding surgeon. This operation and the rare condition of the colon are a part of the Medical History Journal. I am extremely grateful for this life-saving doctor/surgeon. Obviously my work on earth was not completed because my recovery progressed nicely. In fact, after recovery I was able to help my family members in surviving their health problems. The following years were very busy.

In 1980 my dad died and my husband had a stroke the next day. It was very hard to deal with this double trauma. I had guilty feelings because I felt that perhaps there may have been more I could have done for him. Adjusting to the loss of my dad was extremely difficult. A short time after his death I made a suicide attempt but the effort was foiled. When my mind cleared I called Crisis Help Line. In fact, I called them several times. The people on the other end of the phone line listened attentively and advised me to seek medical services. She said,' Suicide is a permanent solution to a temporary problem'. This was hard for me to grasp but I decided to work to get my husband all the therapy that might help him. After two years I suffered physical and mental burnout. Again I called Crisis Help Line and the attentive listener advised medical help to settle me down. My physician advised me to get involved with an activity that I could enjoy at least once a week. So I got involved with a political party that met once a month. This way I met new friends. Then I learned about the Greater Milwaukee Stroke Club. When there were political events I took Steve with me. I attended the Stroke Club to help him meet new people and I became involved with planning and helping with events. Later the Club elected me for their president.

In 1987, my husband died April 15th and my mother died on October 17th of the same year. Now I had no family at all. In my state of mind I reached out for help.

BEGINNING A NEW LIFE ALONE

Suicide again entered my mind- this time I contacted the Psychologist Dr. Gerald Hodan who had helped my husband after the stroke. I would not have been able to continue alone because I had no relatives except I did have some good friends to help me during this trying time.

My sessions with Dr. Gerald Hodan were very helpful in making this gigantic adjustment in my life. Without his excellent professional services, I am sure my life would have been a disaster. He gave me relaxation exercises and various suggestions about reading a travelogue for small trips. Since the time was close to the Christmas holiday Dr. Hodan told me to put up a small tree with my favorite ornaments to help with some pleasant thoughts. He also told me to call him anytime during the season to keep in touch with him. In fact he called me to check up on how I was handling my grief.

In one of the sessions after the holidays he suggested I write a book because he said it would be therapy for me and would be helpful to other people. Upon this idea I wrote and published my first book "See the Rainbow Through the Tears"

The following year 1988 I browsed thru some travel material and decided to plan my vacation. I made a partial payment to insure my reservation to go to Lake Louise and the Banff in Canada. I had seen many travelogues on the Canadian Rockies and looked forward to this vacation. I had a lifelong dream to feast my eyes on this scenery and nearby places of interest. Before I actually went on the trip, I decided to have a physical examination and a mammogram. This test revealed a tumor. A biopsy was performed and it was diagnosed as invasive breast cancer. Dr. Herrington urged me not to delay surgery, but I refused to have surgery until after the Canadian trip I was determined that MY DREAM VACATION WOULD BE A REALITY. The doctor explained the seriousness of invasive breast cancer. My first reaction was denial. I just could not believe the news. I sought a second opinion. Delay of surgery may be putting my life in jeopardy, however at this point my vacation seemed more important. Emotionally, I did not feel I could survive this latest trauma in my life without having this enjoyment that I had planned over a long period of time.

My second opinion came from another reputable physician, Dr. Anthony Sweeney. During the consultation with Dr. Sweeney, he analyzed the film, the slides and endorsed the original diagnosis. He listened patiently as I explained my fears not only of surgery but my concerns about radiation treatments, he then recommended Dr. Marcia Richards, the Director of Radiation Oncology, at the hospital to obtain more information on radiation treatments. She would explain radiation therapy and this would reduce my fears. I made an appointment with Dr. Richards, she answered all my questions, gave me literature and told me she would contact Dr. Herrington and work with him to cure my cancer. I read the literature that night that contained information about the immune system and the effects of stress. After reading this booklet I know why Cancer had attacked me. The previous year with all of the traumas I experienced was very stressful. The stress had caused my cancer because my immune system was weakened. A healthy immune system fights disease. I had experienced a tremendous amount of stress in the prior year in the loss of my family. This planned vacation would relieve me of some stress to help build up my immune system. The literature offered suggestions as to how to build a healthy immune system to aid the body to heal and prevent infection. With my new-found knowledge and ground work in place I could now continue with my   vacation plans to Canada in a carefree manner.

The following paragraph is taken from my notes which were written as I sat by a window as I viewed the splendid scenery.

I am in a cabin at Jasper Park Lodge in Canada. I am on an eight day conducted tour that includes beautiful Lake Louise, the Banff, and the ice fields of the Glaciers and now I am enjoying the majestic mountains outside my window. All the mountains have a personality of their own. Some are snow-capped, others covered with trees of all shapes, sizes, and others have jagged rocks from land-slides. The waterfalls in many places have carved very unusual designs from the force of the volume of water as it tumbles down. These waterfalls are incomprehensible; you would have to see them yourself to appreciate this magnificent sight. This tour included countless attractive sights. We saw beautiful lakes with reflections in the clear green water. It was spectacular! Did I say GREEN water? Yes, the water at Lake Louise and Emerald Lake was an elegant emerald green, caused by some of the elements of the glaciers. We also saw Moraine Lake, which by contrast was a heavenly blue. This also was caused by some of the elements of the glaciers. We had very interesting guides and wonderful people on this tour which added to the pleasure of the trip. I am counting on all the sights and events to help me in the trying days ahead.

Upon completion of my Canadian trip I made arrangements for my operation for breast cancer. I shuddered at the very thought of having surgery. I kept thinking about the nice vacation in Canada as I waited for the day of surgery. I thanked God for the chance to view all that superb scenery. The thoughts of this trip and all the breathtaking beauty helped me daily to reduce the tension of the approaching operation. I was frightened and still found it hard to believe that I was the victim of a new form of grief. There must be a reason, but I consoled myself with the thought that if I cannot find a reason then I must think positive and that a good attitude would increase my chances of a successful survival. My second thought was to try to make some good result from this latest painful event. I came to terms realizing that whatever the out-come; I could still enjoy the beauty of nature and my friends. My friends had urged me not to delay the operation. In the days that followed friends came with flowers, plants and other gifts. My friends were like my family. Indeed, in my opinion, my friends were my family. During the various trying times special people have entered my life. This certainly was true following the loss of my family and my cancer surgery. Wonderful friends have shown concern and family type love. This has given me joy amid my sorrow.

The day before my release from the hospital my doctor smiled as he entered my room to give me the results of the surgery. Dr. Herrington was a skilled surgeon as well as a warm and concerned doctor. He seemed eager and happy to tell me the news I was waiting to hear. He told me that he had removed the lymph nodes under the arm and all the nodes were negative. The good news was that the results were good there also. I was fortunate that the cancer was found in its earliest stages. I was told I would need six weeks of radiation treatments but my hopes for a cure appeared to be very promising. I found from my own experience that there are four things that are necessary to become a survivor:

First...Early detection of Cancer or any other ailment is important.

Second ...Surgery, Radiation or Chemotherapy are all means, of giving hope for survival.

Third... Seek out the very best doctors with whom you can feel confident to trust with your life.

Get a second opinion if you feel more comfortable. Then make the decision.

Fourth ...A positive attitude is essential to improve the emotional and bodily healing. Family support is a great asset. Since I had no family, my loyal friends became my family and gave me this valuable support. To have a positive attitude when faced with a chronic disease or other serious ailment is extremely difficult. With the advances of medical knowledge, complete cures are possible, and good quality of life is attainable. Don't give up HOPE.

After I went home to recuperate, my neighbors, and some of my friends continued to do a number of kind acts and services. Some prepared meals and froze meals for me to use as needed. Some gave me fruit and vegetables and baked chicken. Neighbors volunteered to do shopping and my laundry for me. Others drove me to doctor's offices for appointments.

Sufficient time for healing was allowed and now it was time for radiation treatments. Dr. Richards proceeded to plan my course of treatment and monitored the radiation therapist as to the progress. The radiation therapist had a warm and friendly manner that made me feel relaxed, comfortable and confident that each treatment would go well. He answered my questions and worked closely with Dr. Richards informing her of any problems or questions as he felt appropriate. I have been fortunate to have had these skilled professionals and the excellent care in my fight against cancer. When I started my radiation treatments six weeks seemed a long time so I marked my calendar each day which seemed to help in the count down time. I met many new people while we shared time in the waiting room for our treatments. During those six weeks we had ample time to share our feelings and give support to one another. There is no guarantee that cancer will not appear again, but I have today to enjoy and today to make a few more of my dreams become realities.

I was very depressed in the beginning when I first heard that I had this dreaded disease. I still have my low moments but I have again made visits to my psychologist, Dr. Hodan. During the sessions he asked me what my thoughts were and how this helped me to cope. He thought the method I used was very good and that perhaps I should write a book to help others. During one of my sessions in 1988 he encourage me to pursue writing the book in fact each session he would ask me questions about the progress .This was an incentive to help me complete the project and I was successful in having it published in 1990. The book was another way to help others for I have a better under-standing of pain and suffering of other people. Furthermore, in my search for a kind loving God, I found His love came to me through the many good people who showed their kindness, concern and love for me. I have been the recipient of a great deal of love and kindness. It seems strange but it's true, that often a person in suffering can find wisdom and strength.

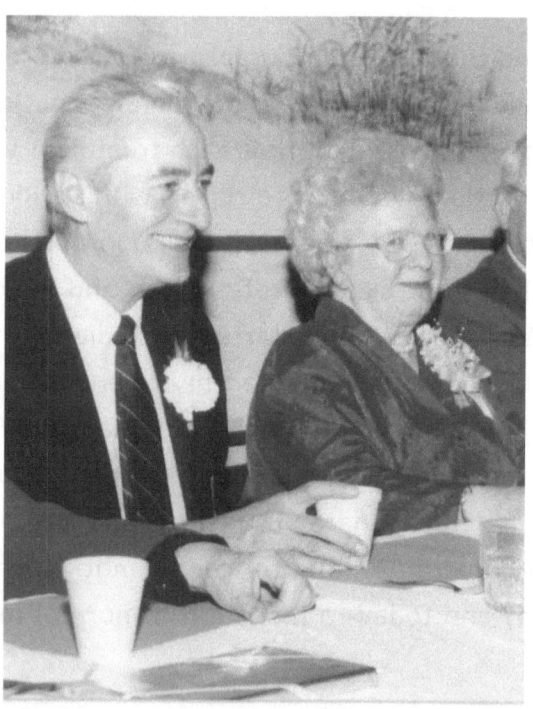

Dr. Gerald Hodan Psychologist at my dinner

When I published my first book

I mentioned earlier about my involvement with the Stroke Club during the years my husband was a member of the club. I had been elected president of the Club after my husband died, and prior to my learning that I had cancer. I wanted to withdraw my nomination to be president. My request was voted down by a unanimous decision. I was told, "We need you and you need us. We will help you but we want you to be our president. You are setting a precedent because all former officers were stroke survivors. We will be proud to have you as our leader. We understand and we care." What a wonderful group of people to make all these kind remarks. After hearing these comments those words of encouragements I resolved that there was no choice but to accept this honor being bestowed on me. It gave me a greater incentive to recover so I could be an active president of the Stroke Club. That night I began to make a comparison between my chronic ailment and those who have to live with the effects of a stroke. When you are paralyzed by a stroke you know you will have to adjust the best you can because there is no end to your condition. You go on living and facing the challenges of every day. Cancer is called a chronic ailment because you may or may not be cured. You live each day with the need to try to keep it under control, and hopefully to have a cure, but you do not know of the hidden activity of the disease.

So in reality I am one with my Stroke Club friends because we share a chronic ailment. I may not have a stroke but I have a disease that is just as threatening, critical and of a similar challenge. Sometimes I feel that maybe one of the reasons for my cancer is so that I can relate more closely to and help even more people in my life. I had searched for some reason to accept this new traumatic event in my life. I think I found that reason and this thought brings some comfort to me. I have hope for today and even greater hope for a good tomorrow. Hope is a very important element in everyone's life. My goal is not only to survive but to live a healthy and productive life, for as long as possible. Search for a meaning for your life and go for it! This is my way of going on with life. I am a very active president of the Stroke Club. I enjoy all the activities with the members and their families.

My mother once told me that a person must work as if everything depended on you and then pray as if everything depended on God. To me surgery scars are battle scars. You know you were in a fight but you survived. After survival the next fight is to try and appreciate each day and to obtain from each day as much happiness as possible. In moments of solitude my mind has flashed back to past happy events.

My health conditions seem stabilized now. I have been active and become involved helping people in various ways and will continue to do so as long as possible. I am looking forward to some personal pleasures in my life. My husband and I saved for our retirement years, but he did not live to fulfill his dreams. A short time before his last stroke he expressed to me his wishes that I take care of myself and enjoy my life.

Another suggestion of Dr. Hodan was to take up a new hobby. That appealed to me. I always liked music and dancing. So I started taking ballroom dance lessons. So with dancing and travel as objections I started to build my life.

Travel is an excellent way to develop new friendships, as well as to enjoy my established family of friends. My major depressions have diminished. There are still days in my life which have clouds of sadness, but I try to look beyond to see the sun and a brighter tomorrow. Most people, (myself included) have Peaks and Valleys in their life. The Peaks are the joyous times and the Valleys occur when illness and accidents happen. This is the time you use the memories of pleasant events to aid in your recovery. I call this the positive attitude of HOPE. Life is not going to be a bed of roses. There are far too many thorns in the form of pain and suffering. However, like the beauty of the rose there is happiness to be found in life. Happiness is whatever appeals to the individual but we sometimes have to take time out to find how to tap that source of happiness and restore the desire to live and enjoy. Even in my solitude, I sense the continuing love of Steve and my parents and feel through my memory of them that they too are enjoying the fullness of my living which I have now. I have learned a valuable lesson since I live alone. I have cried many times and found that tears are a part of the healing process. Bottled up grief not only prolongs grief but can also cause serious health problems. Since there are many people who live alone as I do, loneliness can lead to depression.

In addition to the help from my psychologist, I have developed a few things that help me. I enjoy eating at a restaurant and say a few kind words to waitresses; I buy myself some flowers once in a while and call up a friend to ask what is new in their life. I play some old records or watch a video. Not everyone has these assets but the library will mail books to people who have difficulty reading but you need someone to obtain a library card for you. Hope some of these ideas will help the reader.

When I look back on my sorrows and trials it seems a small miracle that I am able to evaluate the knowledge gained through these experiences. I know my suicide attempts were really a cry for help. People use suicide attempts to get help which many need at some time in their life, when faced with burdens of pain, grief or separation from loved ones. When I called the Crisis help line the person would listen to me and then say my problems are temporary.

Think about how you can change your conditions and share your thoughts with others by joining a support group to help find an answer, suicide is permanent. I am grateful to those unknown people who patiently listened to me, when at that time of my life I knew of no other place to turn. I was fortunate to have reached out for help before it was too late. Men and women attend support groups, because people have experienced similar trials. Men seldom have a place to release their thought and feelings. Sadness is a human emotion. The need to reveal this emotion is as important, to men as well as women. In my first book I spent many hours setting forth my ideas of how I dealt with grief. This chapter received many favorable comments so it is incorporated here.

In summary it may be worthwhile to use a key word when you are confronted with grief or with a chronic ailment. The word is **STOPS** covers a few hints which may prove useful in surviving depression.

S ....Seek out support groups in time of grief. When confronted with a chronic ailment ask your doctor or hospital staff to refer you to a support group. That concerns you or one of your family members.

T ....Tears are a means of setting free emotions of sadness and will help in the healing process.

O ....One day at a time is enough to handle. Today may seem extremely hard but tomorrow may be better.

P..... Prescription drugs may be beneficial during the period of initial shock. Psychologists and in some cases other professionals can assist you in making adjustments in your life. Even a very understanding friend may be a great help.

S.....Suicide is a permanent solution to a temporary problem. Every problem has an answer.

Be willing to ASK FOR HELP from other people! Don't Throw In The Towel!

My first book "See the Rainbow through the Tears" is no longer available.

A NEW YEAR A NEW HOPE

I approached 1989 with an optimistic attitude. I had survived the pain of radiation in an attempt to cure my cancer. I had some enjoyment in my Canada tour. New plans would be a conducted tour to Alaska July 5th to the 18th 1989, to get a little relaxation. The tour was mostly by boat and some bus scenery. The Glaciers are a remainder of the ice ages. At times huge chunks of ice break off and form a bay of water and many of these giant pieces float in water. It is a common sight to see a mother seal and her pup on these icebergs. Whales feed in these waters also. This is only a part of the amazing scenery. There were helicopter tours over the Mendenhall Glacier that took people over the tops of these awesome mountains of ice. I gathered enough courage to take this helicopter ride. The vehicle could only take five passengers at a time plus the pilot. Each person had to be weighed for proper balance. Two people in the back seats, two people in the front and I was put in the middle as a light weight. It is difficult to describe the unusual beautiful blue color that appeared to be water between these mountains of ice. The beauty was a distraction from any anxiety I felt on that ride which I never expected to partake. The bus trips were interesting too. I will relate a little incident experienced while waiting for our bus to arrive for a scenic tour. We were at a bar having refreshments, and while drinking my beverage I somehow spilled it on my new blouse. The blouse had a picture of Mt. McKinley and nearby glaciers on it. I felt embarrassed and exclaimed "I have just had a glacier melt!" It made everyone laugh, especially since the water was in the middle of my chest where Mt McKinley was shown. Even after the trip people were joking about the incident.

The bus trip to Denali National Park from Fairbanks was a 70 mile bus ride on dirt roads. The scenery was nice and we saw many animals such as moose, goats, white sheep and bears. The bus was parked at a point where we could have a clear view of Mt McKinley, which is the tallest peak of the mountains in North America. We were given time to walk around the area but we were cautioned not to eat any food while outside the bus because the bears could cause us trouble. Since Alaska is 1/5 the size of United States and Mt McKinley is in the center of the state, we knew that there would be many other interesting sights to be seen.

The next day we again would be taking the cruise ship through the southeastern inner passage. The Cruise ship "Discovery" had three decks and was like a floating resort. The Captain would give a narrative about the various cities and in some cases we would have a chance to go onto the land, for some sightseeing or to stay on the land for a night or two before boarding the cruise ship again.

The next stop on the tour was Juneau, the State Capitol, a modern city with gift shops and a popular tavern called the Red Dog Saloon. No tours in this place. From this short stop in Juneau our bus came to take us to the ice fields. The major point of interest was the ice fields. We were told to dress warmer because we would be in an open vehicle and would be permitted to walk on the ice. There were some crevasses where you could see clear blue water. The guide mentioned that this mountain of ice was shrinking and that perhaps in time this type of trip would not be possible.

Matanuska Valley was a bus ride to the farmlands. Not just ordinary farms because Alaska has a growing season that is 120 days long and the produce are extra-large. Example: a large tomato is like an oversized small pumpkin. The example just mentioned seems unbelievable but I did order a tomato stuffed with delicious chicken salad for lunch one day that was a whole meal with no room for dessert. The next part of the travel was on the passenger cruise ship and the Captain would nar-rate information about the cities we were viewing. Ketchikan is the 4th largest city with the homes built on the hillside. It is about 2 blocks long and five miles wide. It is noted as a fishing port. The National Park in this area has numerous Indian totem poles. .Sitka, formerly the capitol, is now a national park. St. Nicholas Russian Church, built in 1867, is a historical museum. In 1916, the Pioneer Home for the elderly was built for residents who lived in Alaska 15 years or more. It had three floors and a space about a quarter of a block long.

Skagway is a National Park established and maintained as close a replica of the gold rush days   in 1894 including the store fronts and the Klondike Inn where part of the lawlessness is reenacted in shows. We also had a short bus ride to view the graves of some of the outlaws of that time. The hotel we stayed at had good food but no TV and no telephones. A wake up call in the morning was a loud knock on the door. Even a chance to pan for gold (not much) turned out to be just enough to see with a magnifying glass. We even had a chance to see the gigantic 800 miles pipeline built from Fairbanks to Valdez to move what was called 'black gold'.

Anchorage experienced an earthquake on Good Friday in 1964, the damage was tremendous. There is a building with a program that tells details about the damage and the seats rumble under a person to give a small example of the feeling at the time. This is known as Earthquake Park. We stayed at the beautiful modern Anchorage Hotel with an exquisite dining room on the top level of the hotel. The food was elegant and the music was very delightful. It was also amazing to stand out on the balcony at 2:30 a.m. and take pictures of the city. It felt strange to go to bed at night with brightness equivalent to dusk at early evening. Every part of this Alaska trip was an adventure. Even opening the door to your room with a card instead of a key was new to me. When Alaska was purchased from Russia in 1867, people called it "Seward's ice box". Little did they know the value of this great land?

Arriving home after a relaxing scenic and interesting Alaska vacation, my thoughts were directed to new ventures. My first book was published and I had interviews with a few newspapers, some speaking-engagements on the local radio station WTMJ, interviews on LocalTV Channel 12 and a ½ hour visit on a local cable show. All these events were exciting to me. Favorable comments received made me happy to have helped other people.

I also began taking Ballroom Dance Lessons in 1990. All of these new adventures opened up a brand new world to me. In a short time, various small dance competitions were held in which I participated. The most exciting competition was scheduled at the Holiday Inn in Las Vegas Nevada on February 2, 1992. This was special. It was called the challenge of champions. I won three medals for some dances.   My solo dance with my teacher, to the "moon river" melody, required special acting to illustrate the words.   I won a beautiful 17 inch tall trophy for this solo dance with my teacher for this performance.   When they scanned my luggage at the airport they thought this trophy was a weapon . When I arrived home I found my face powder had opened and was spread all over my clothes.   I figured my bag had been searched.

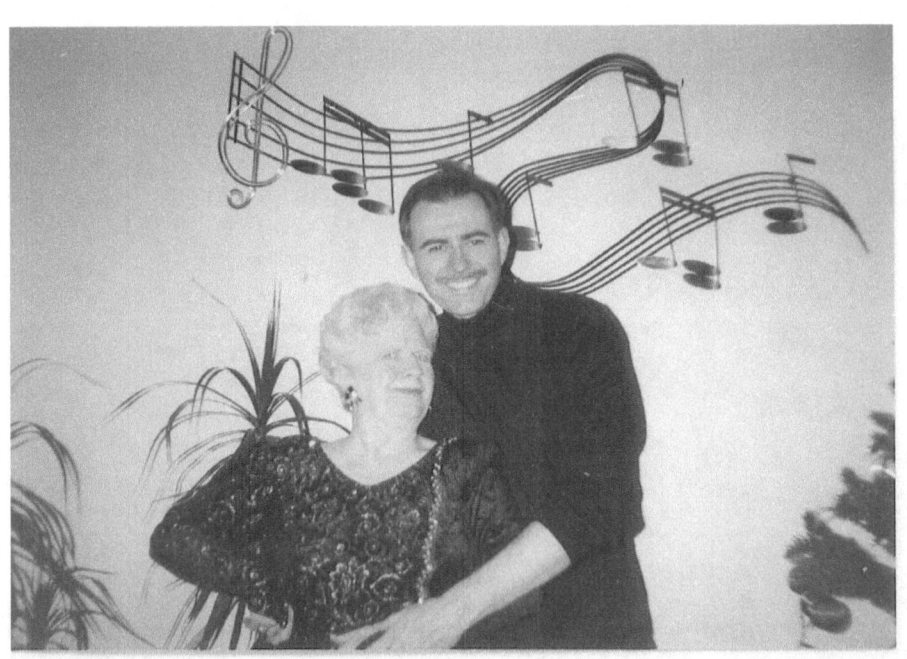

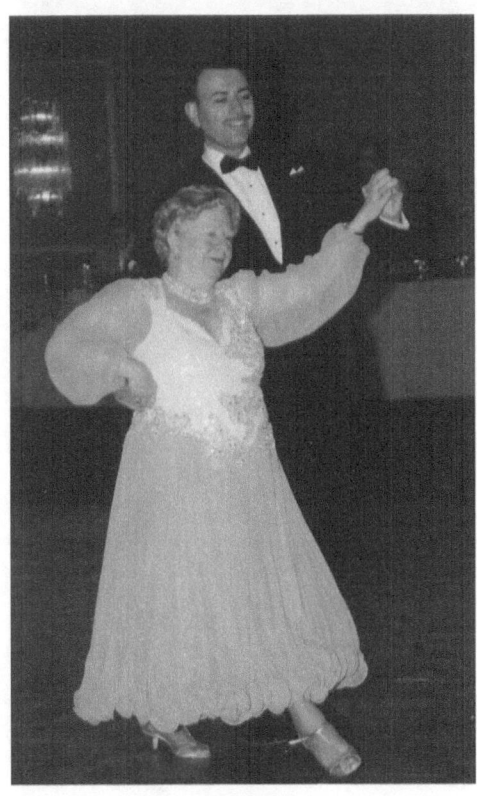

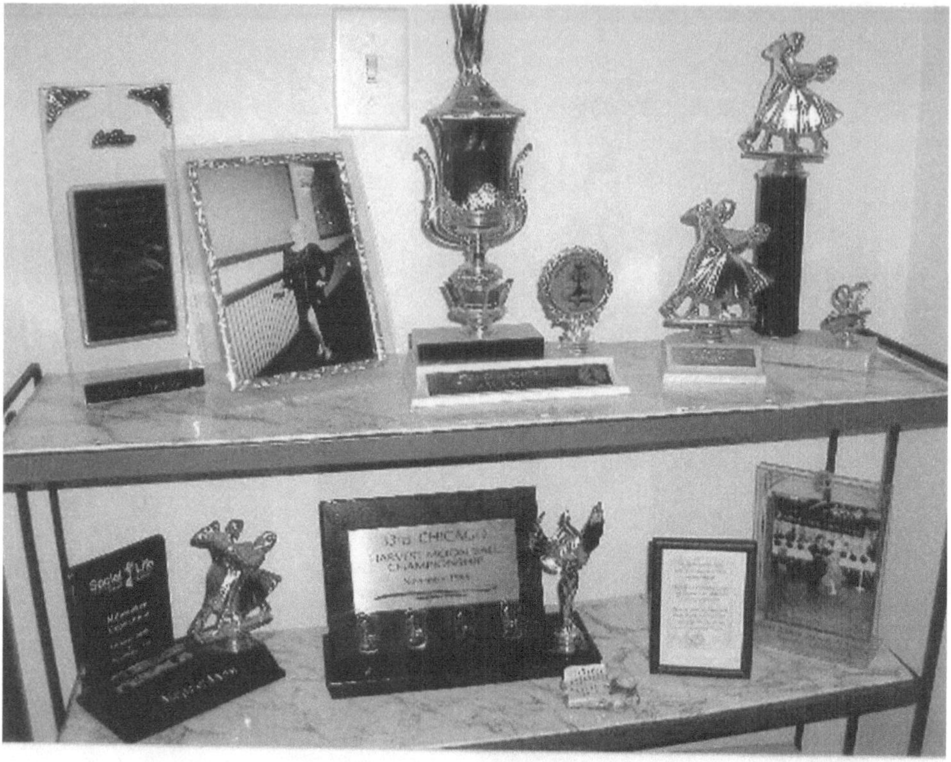

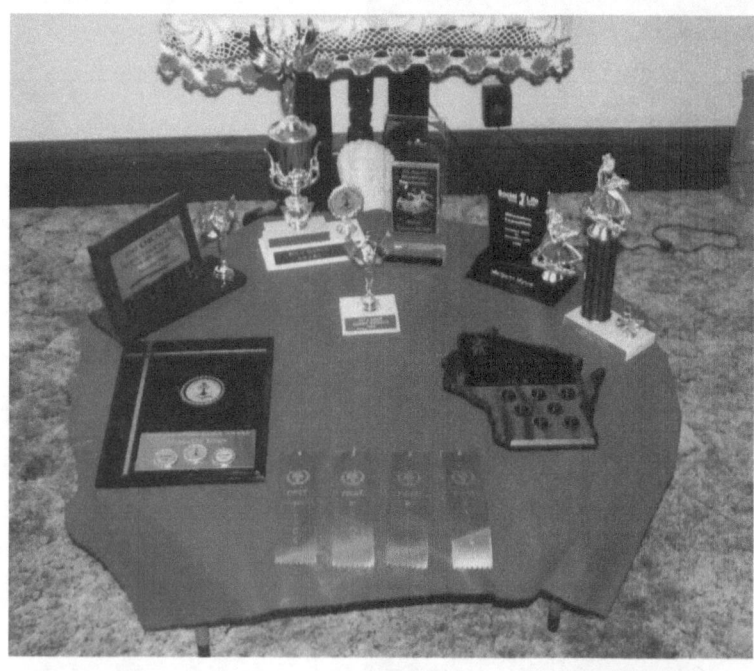

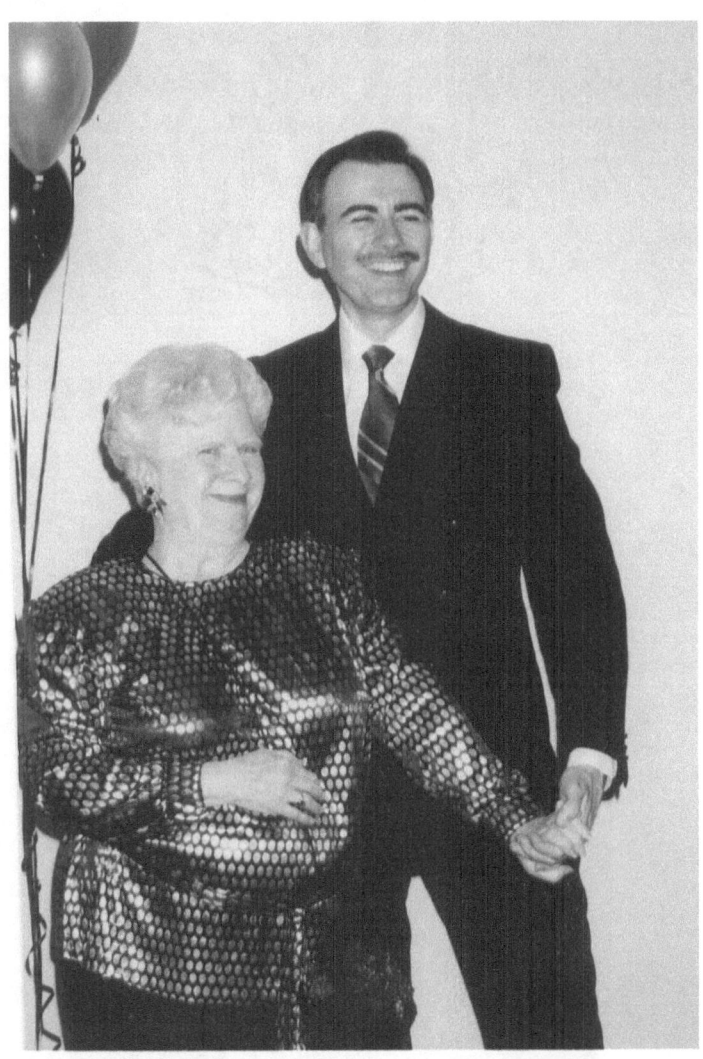

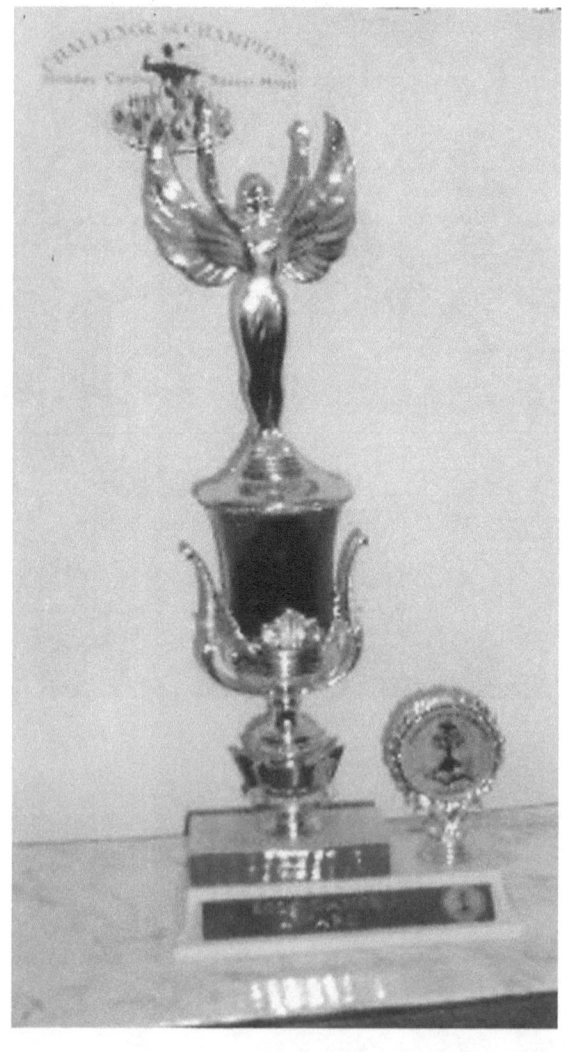

BEAUTIFUL HAWAII

A special tour began April 7, 1994, to beautiful Hawaii. My travel companion was a Nun named Sister Leora. Nuns always travel with a companion and Sister Leora had to obtain special permission to travel with me. We visited four islands in Hawaii, Oahu, Maui, Kona and Kauai. We were amazed by the beauty of the Waimea Canyon, which is known as the "Grand Canyon of the Pacific" and is located in Kauai. Kauai has beautiful dense tropical growth in the Fern Grotto. It is rightly called the "Garden Isle". People at various times sing songs that echo over the land. Before we left this island we had lunch at the luxurious Coco-Palms Resort that was set on 45 acres of secluded coconut grove. On this same property was the Immaculate Conception Church, where many visitors are married and have their receptions at this remarkably beautiful place.

Kona is unique in having a glass-bottom boat and watching divers feeding fish to bring them close to the windows for the passengers to see them.

In Honolulu, we were taken to see the U.S.S. Arizona Memorial, where so many of our servicemen are buried as a result of the Pearl Harbor bombing. It is quite a sight and it makes me feel sad, even today, as I recall this part of the trip. Maui is called the 'Garden isle' because this island has a large variety of many beautiful flowers. There are active and inactive volcanoes. The Haleakala Crater is known to be an active volcano.

The following year, in the summer of 1995, I took a conducted tour to visit the Grand Canyon in Colorado. On this trip I met Mona Slaney, her daughter Patricia and her fiancé Victor Medina. They said they would love to invite me to their wedding that was to be held the next year. They were from the state of Massachusetts. The entire trip was enjoyable, and afterwards Ms. Slaney and I would become good pen-pals. When I returned from this trip I prepared for a dance competition that was to be held in October, 1995 at the Social Life Dance Studio in Waukesha. This was a fun night as it was not only a dance competition but also a costume Halloween Party. This party was a great ending to a wonderful year.

ANOTHER SETBACK

March 1996 I had a Cancer return, this time in the right breast. This surgery was considered very serious, because it was a six month fast growing tumor. After surgery I had to take occupational therapy to gain the use of my arm because the surgeon made an error and cut a nerve or tendon which caused a displaced tendon under the armpit. The therapy lasted until June, and my sessions with Radiation began. I had very strong Radiation for six weeks. The burn was so severe that medication had to be applied daily to keep the skin from breaking. There were times when the skin broke in the beginning but the medicine did heal the burned breast. The Radiation was extremely painful because of the injury that occurred in surgery as well as the treatment itself. In the meantime I did receive a wedding invitation from Pat and Victor to attend their wedding on September 28, 1996 in Needham, Mass. The healing was sufficient for me to look forward to their wedding. I was greeted at the airport and reservations were made for me to stay overnight at the Wellesley Inn which was a very old and famous place. The bed reminded me of the George Washington era, when the beds were high off the floor and had a canopy above. I had to use a stool to climb up to get in bed. Wellesley Inn is near Wellesley College, which was a place for families to stay when visiting their children. This historic place has since been dismantled.

This has been a year of pain and joy and even after the beautiful wedding, the tour I took, and meeting nice people there was one more fantastic event. On Nov 29th & 30th, I participated in the Chicago Harvest Ballroom Competition. The plaque I received meant a great deal after all the events of the year.

When I attended the wedding during the last year, Mona, the mother of the bride, mentioned she would like to visit Canada, and especially the Calgary Stampede. We talked about making plans with the same travel agency for a tour where we would meet at a given point so we could finish the flight together on the same airline to make this two-some possible. Plans were successfully made, so on June 30, 1997 Mona Slaney and I began our tour. The EAST-WEST Travel Agency sent each of us an itinerary that covered all the places of interest from June 30th to July 11.1997. We both wanted to go to Calgary, Canada to see a special horse show and we wanted to see the red coat mounted police. The tour did this and more as you will soon read.

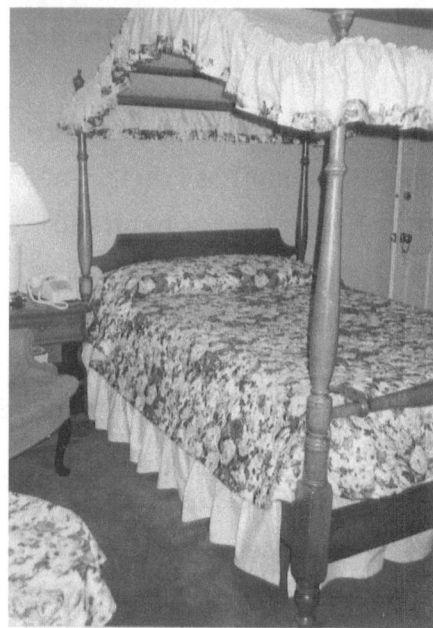

Bed at Wellsley Inn 9-28-96

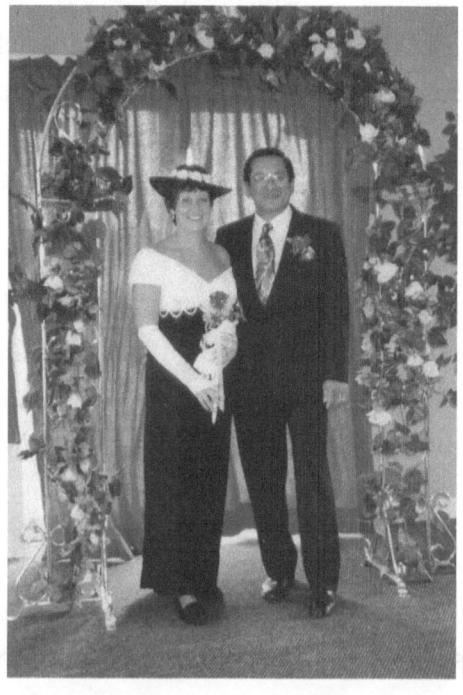

Pat & Victor Wedding

9-28-96

VANCOUVER

On June 30, 1997 Mona Slaney and I met at Seattle to begin our trip together. The next day we boarded a cruise ship to Vancouver, B.C. Upon landing we had a sight-seeing trip to Stanley Park to look at the Bloedel Conservatory, where beautiful flowers can be seen year-round. The next place was the Gaston Mall to see a steam-powered clock, with time to shop and get a little lunch. Later, we checked into our lodging at Chateau Victoria. The next day we went to the beautiful Buchart Gardens, where 50 acres of land contains a multitude of individual gardens. There is the Japanese Garden, with a red bridge over a waterfall and ponds with floating flowers, a rustic tea house that was surrounded by rhododendrons and Japanese maple trees. There also is an Italian Garden that has a mermaid fountain surrounded with geraniums, coreopsis, and pink snapdragons with archways and benches. These are only two examples of the six outstanding gardens we saw. Each set of gardens has a specialty. There are tuberous begonias and fuchsias that are large and colorful as you continue along the pathways. The trees are shaped in multiple ways and cement benches and statues complement the view.

The next day was July 4th and we went to the Rockies National Parks. Yoho National Park contains a beautiful lake called Emerald Lake because of its clear green water. The glacial melt water feeding the lake contains fine silt which stays suspended in the water reflecting the green rays of this lake. The same condition causes Lake Louise to have this same beautiful color. Tonight our lodging will be at Chateau Lake Louise.

Today is Saturday and is a Leisure Day for Hikes and Pictures. Mona Slaney and I decided to take the long walk that surrounds the Lake. The length of the lake is one and a half miles. We walked about a mile. We knew we had to walk back to the Lodge and we felt we should save ourselves for the next day. We took pictures of people in boats and we took

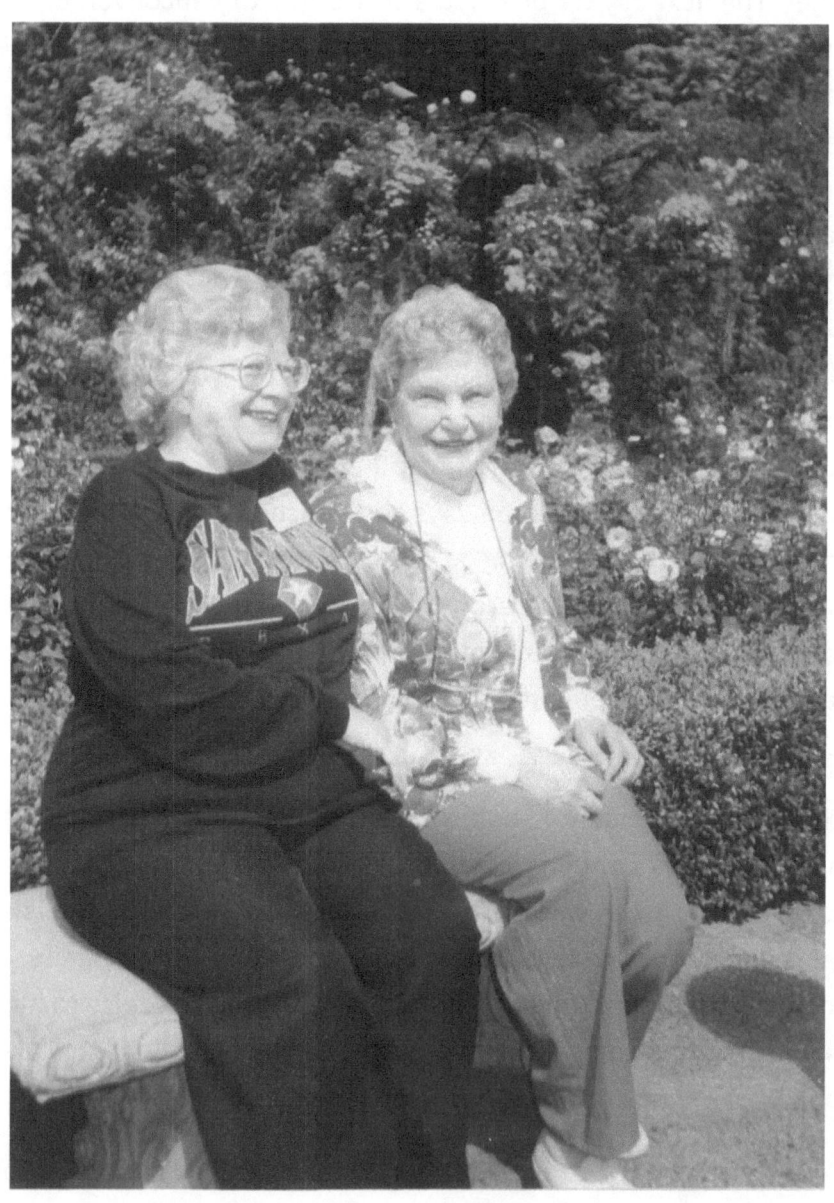

a picture of each other on this extra-long walk. Some people took horse rides up the hill to attempt to climb Mt Victoria but we did not walk that far. Today the sun was bright and reflected on the lake displaying the clear opaque turquoise water. That night there was a severe storm. Most lights went out and our wing was the only one with a dim light. Over the loud speaker we were told not to go out of our rooms. I looked out the window and the Lake was jet black. With a surge of lighting was the outline of the mountain. Whenever I went on a trip after this experience I always take a flashlight. The next morning we were traveling again.

Peyto Glacier is located along the ice fields in Banff National Park in the foreground is Peyto Lake that was very unusual because it was shaped like three pointed fingers. I stood on a ledge to take a picture of it. When I got home I saw a large painting in an art store, bought it and is now displayed in my home. There were other stopping points to take pictures as we traveled on to Bow Lake and the Athabasca Falls. Lodging tonight was the Sawridge Hotel in Jasper, and travel today will include a delightful hour and a half scenic narrated cruise on Maligne Lake. The boat is fully enclosed and heated, and staffed by Coast Guard licensed crew members. This lake is the second largest glacial lake in the world; it is 14 miles in length, the deepest part is 319 ft., and the lowest part is 150 ft. I wrote notes on the trip to keep with the pictures. I knew I would not remember all the data without my notes. The highlight of today will be to the Columbia Ice Fields. There is a special equipped vehicle called the Snow Coach that will take us on the tour up the snow covered Athabasca Glacier. We were taken up to the elevation of 7000 ft., which was the turnaround point at which we were permitted to get off the bus and to walk on the ice. We had been told to wear warm clothes and we now knew the reason. There were crevasses (cracks in the ice) in several places in the ice. Some were wide enough to see clear water. People took chances to try to scoop up to drink the water which they said was the best ever tasted. The guide told us that the ice field was

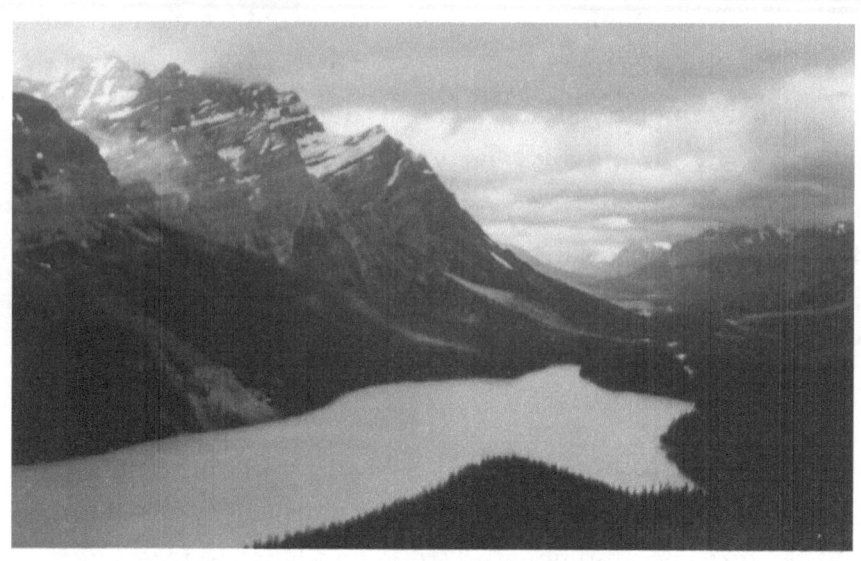

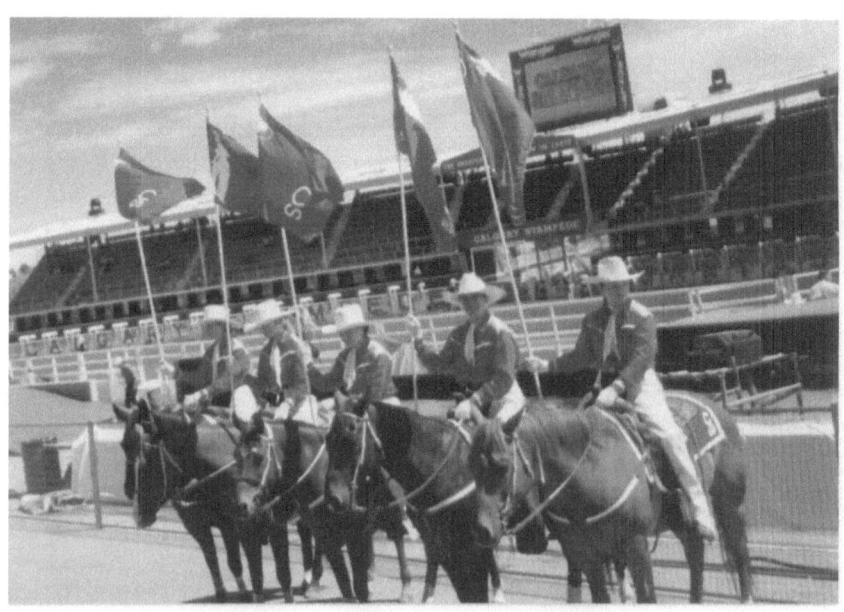

melting at a slow pace but there may be a time when this ride may not be available. The lodging tonight is at the Banff Hotel. Today is the last day of this tour. We anxiously looked forward to the day's big event, the Calgary Stampede. The large grandstand was filled to capacity but our Group Tour Coordinators Ellen & Vince Lanzalotta did splendid planning to obtain excellent seating for us to view this spectacular event. The horses were magnificent animals and their riders did bare back tricks some riders did lasso and roping of cows as would be expected in a rodeo. There were chuck wagon races and horse racing. Each element seemed to outdo the previous performance. The costumes were very colorful too. This certainly was an outstanding event. We wanted to see the Mounted Police in their red uniforms and we did. Lodging tonight will be the Holiday Inn and we will have an early start for our trip home. We had a wonderful vacation. We may not have another opportunity to do a vacation again but our friendship is solid and we will keep it alive and well by phone and letters.

In August of 1997, I broke my wrist and arm in 9 places, so I had very little activity the remainder of the year. In the middle part of 1998 my dancing instructor helped me to resume taking dance lessons. But by September I had cataract surgery in my right eye and in November, another cataract surgery in the left eye. 1999 was off to another bad start, and in February, Pneumonia, a bronchial infection and Congestive Heart Failure tore me apart. After surviving this bad start it was time to turn things around. I saw tour literature about the Columbia River Gorge scheduled for June 10th thru June 15th. This was only six days and promised to be very relaxing. The first bus stop would be the Portland Rose Society's Spring Rose Show, where everyone was anxious to take pictures. We stayed at the Ramada Plaza Hotel, with its full service restaurant and enjoyable evening dinner. Each day had different entertainment planned and gorgeous scenery to observe. There was a Festival of Bands competition with over 500 members of all ages. The Grand Floral Parade of Floats which contained beautiful arrangements of flowers. On

the bus tour we were informed that the Columbia River Gorge is between two states; Washington and Oregon. Near the western end of the
Gorge is the modern city of Portland, Oregon. During the ride we saw
numerous waterfalls--the most breathtaking sight was the Multnomah
Falls that is the 2nd highest waterfall in the U.S. The water falls from 620
feet in a series of basins carved by the water. This was a camera person's dream sight. Today was filled with falls and mountains with special charm and beauty. Arriving back at the hotel we had a nice dinner
and leisure visit.

The last day of our tour was the Mt. St. Helen visitor center where
pictures revealed some of the awesome volcanic devastation that occurred previously on May 18, 1980. Mt. St Helen was 9,677 feet at the
time of eruption and it became a cloud of ash and volcanic debris rising
to 60,000 feet, burying homes and people and changing the landscape
within a few minutes. Now this mountain stands at 8,363 feet. Native
Americans call it "Fire Mountain". The scenery looks strangely peaceful
now. People made comments about the variety of this trip as our bus
headed to our original starting point of our homes.

TURNING POINT IN MY LIFE

In the year 2000 I made the biggest mistake in my life. I altered my life from that date until now. I sold my home! There were so many so-called friends that were constantly telling me that the house was too much to care for, especially shoveling snow and cutting grass. I hired people when necessary. Even one of the doctors thought it was a good idea because I had stairs to climb and there would be the danger of falling. I was active in the neighborhood. I was a Block Watch Captain and I took up a collection for snow removal in the alley in the winter, since it was very steep and cars found it difficult to manage. The house was in great condition .The Bathroom had been remodeled and a Recreation room built just a short time before my parents died. The house sold fast. I moved to a retirement community... another big mistake. In the process of moving in I was robbed of a large sum of money. I was told later that there had been other robberies and that a cleaning lady employee had been caught in the act in one instance. However, I never recovered any of my money. The people who prodded me into the situation of selling my home, (Yes, you guessed it) disappeared.

After I got settled I resumed my dancing lessons, I made some new friends. After I dried my tears, I tried to reclaim my life again It would take a while but two years later I took a trip.

On September 14, 2002 I took a bus tour to New York because it included the Baseball Hall of Fame. It was exciting to view all the memorabilia of those great baseball players of the past, especially my favorite player Lou Gehrig. There were many other sights of interests.

2003 The tour was to Branson, Missouri often referred to as the "Music Show Capital of the World!" The tour included seeing Andy Williams with many talented performers... Shoji Tabuchi, a classical violinist who also played country western music, had numerous entertainers including his own wife performing with him. The background was colorful, ar-

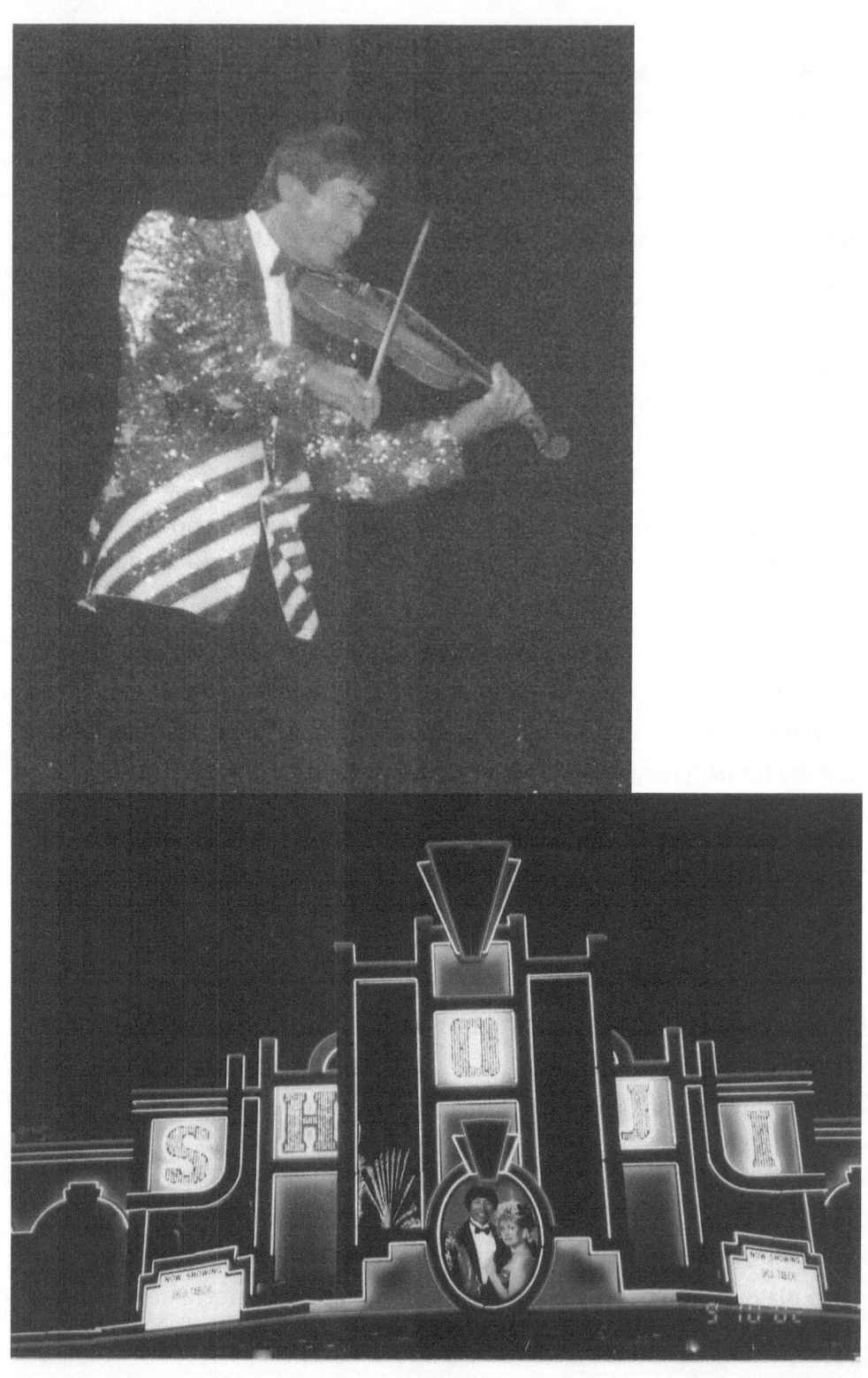

tistic and a quality befitting the talented performer. The show place itself was elegant including the bathrooms with flowers, perfumes and special soaps and gold faucets. The Russian Comedian Yakov Smirnoff was very humorous and yet had a very tasteful way of comparing his homeland Russia with life in the United States. He expressed his gratitude to those who helped him as an immigrant and declared his patriotism to his new country. His closing act was a sincere tribute to the United States. The Showboat called the Branson Bell was a scenic boat ride that had a lovely stage show and a delicious meal.

Later that evening we had dinner at a rustic type of place that had a stage show called the Dinette and Pump Boys. The show was a nice comedy and the meal served was very tasty chicken. Before this tour ended we also heard Frederick and his magic pianos. This was very colorful with dancing waters in the background with colorful lights that responded to the notes played on the piano. The grand finale was when two pianos moved simultaneously to the center of the stage and Frederick played both pianos - one with each hand. The next day this fabulous vacation came to a close.

After my Branson vacation I began taking dance lessons again. There were no competitions scheduled for the remaining part of 2003, so my teacher thought it would be nice to put on a program of dance for older people. There were senior residences in the area that might enjoy a program of dance entertainment. I agreed to be his partner to illustrate many varieties of both Waltzes, Fox Trots, Tango, Rumba Samba and a large selection of other dances. So on October 19th we performed and it was well accepted.

In 2004 I spent some time doing political campaigning again which I had not done since my husband died.

THE TURBULENT YEARS

The Turbulent years of 2005 and 2006 would be the most difficult years to survive because of the remaining pain, scars and memories. The shock was made somewhat easier because of established friends and new people that entered my life. In 2005 I had a very serious fall causing multiple injuries. The day started nice with a delicious meal at Red Lobster Restaurant. The seafood was very tasty but they serve cheese muffins and I do not like to waste food. I asked the waitress to take them back because I am highly allergic to cheese. She suggested taking them along and giving them to friends. Good idea? When I arrived home I took them to a neighbor. I do not know if I tripped on some object or lost balance? I fell to the ground and could not get up... At the hospital I was told that my injuries were a torn rotary cuff, sprained ankle, back injury and numerous bruises. A GOOD DEED WITH BAD RESULTS! I had severe pain, several doctor bills and several weeks of intense physical therapy.

The next year, 2006, would be best expressed as being put on trial for test endurance. The year stated good. I recovered from my injuries and was back dancing again. A program was being planned for Wednesday April 19th which would have celebrities as well as teachers and students from various studios. It would be a local version of Dancing with the Stars. I was excited knowing that Melodie Wilson from Channel 4 would be one of the celebrity dancers. She was both charming and graceful as I knew she would be from seeing her on the television news show. Two days later, April 21st, my dancing instructor Cary Zeugner, was killed by a drunk driver who was also a drug abuser. The speeding driver ran a red light to avoid the police car that was pursuing him. He hit Cary's car with terrific force that knocked down the light pole and killed him instantly. That night Cary was driving to the studio to teach a dancing class. Cary's death on April 21, 2006 was a great loss to the community and to all who knew him. Cary was very active in church work. He had a beautiful voice and sang in the choir. He was helpful to anyone who needed a task that he could do. His main job was that of an electrician. He helped me with many of my household problems: such as putting up my Christmas tree, moving some furniture, and many other tasks that I was not able to do. He was more than a good dance instructor; he was a true friend to me and to everyone who knew him. The loss of my dance instructor is a painful memory. The place where he was killed by that drunk driver is near my home and each day I drive by it is a constant reminder of this tragedy.

It is no surprise that this stress lowered my immune System and caused cancer to return with vengeance. Dr. Gregory Ekbom, a surgeon and specialist in vascular surgery and comprehensive breast care reviewed my mammogram .He advised me that this cancer was more serious than my previous bouts with cancer. This was Infiltrating Ductile Cancer which required a Mastectomy. Dr. Ekbom explained the necessity of this radical surgery and then to soften the blow prayed with me. The surgery was November 30th 2006 and this caring surgeon monitored the recovery period frequently and prescribed therapy to regain strength and prevent lymphoma. I have been fortunate to have had good competent doctors with my encounters with cancer. The following year was absorbed mostly by treatments and therapy. Recovery took a long time as well as adjusting to the loss of part of my body. I felt like I was half a woman, even though I could use a pad to make my clothes fit better. I knew my thinking about this also had to change in order to look at the brighter side of my survival. I had compassion for others when they lost a breast, eyesight, a limb or other major disability and even a greater appreciation for the sacrifice of people serving in the military.

Now I must adjust to my loss. I realized that to improve my health I would like to have a change of scenery. So August 20, 2007, I made plans for a tour to the Shenandoah Valley, in Virginia. I was not able to travel alone, so I asked a retired nurse Dorothy Oldham to accompany me. To reach the Caverns it would be a 105 mile skyline drive, which on a clear day would have given us a nice view of the Blue Ridge Mountains. The colorful green valley could not be seen so on this trip we had to settle for a postcard because today the driver could barely see the road. The Shenandoah Caverns were spectacular. The elevator took us down to the ground floor which consisted of small and large stones which made it difficult to walk on. Then caution had to be taken because the Stalagmite formations which are icicle shaped deposits on the cavern floor. We also had to be careful of the Stalactite which are icicle shaped deposits hanging from the ceiling. These formations were so unusual and attractive that if you were not aware of either type, in a given moment a person could be seriously hurt. I was glad Dorothy was with me to make me alert to possible dangers. She also helped me in managing my walker in these conditions. The most unusual Stalactite had the appearance of stripes of bacon. We were told that this was pictured in the National Geographic Magazine. There were many other rare formations.

Other sights of interest included visiting homes of famous people such as former presidents Thomas Jefferson, James Madison and Woodrow Wilson, just to name a few. We also saw replicas of some of the Civil War Battles, museums, and many other historic places. Along the driveways were pretty wild flowers, birds, butterflies, deer and waterfalls. So in the midst of so many trials there is also a great deal of beauty. Homeward bound I wondered what the future would hold given my health conditions. God had given me strength to survive so many serious surgeries and trials so I will value and use each day that is given to me in the most reasonable way.

My health seemed good but on August 5, 2008 Cancer appeared again. Two lumps this time, one on the incision of the mastectomy and one on the breast bone. Now I thought there would be nothing more to plan for my life. I would just try to help other people whenever possible and enjoy each day in a simple way. Then the unexpected happened! I knew a family for many years who had a tragedy happen to one of their children and I thought maybe I might help them in some way. Their little girl almost died in a lake accident. She did survive after being in the hospital for several weeks I visited her in the hospital and watched as she improved. She received many gifts from friends and relatives that were articles pertaining to Disney World characters. Her dad said he promised that someday he would take her there. I knew there would be no more traveling for me, so I offered the family a chance for the trip. I still had some savings in the bank but the parents did not want to accept it especially when they found out I did not intend to go with them. I did not want to be a burden to them. The father said wheelchairs are available at Disney World and he would gladly push me and help with any entertainment ride I would like to go on. His older two sons said they would alternate and help push the wheelchair also. The parents were going to drive their van and to help with expense they would make sandwiches and some cooked meals to take along in the ice cooler. Advanced planning we were able to rent a home with five bedrooms. Residents of Florida have a company to handle renting their homes to vacationers. I sent the money for the rent of the home and the tickets for the Disney rides and events. So in August 2009 the opportunity was possible for a vacation I did not expect to have due to all my health problems. I enjoyed the fun rides with the children. The Small World boat ride with scenery and music was very enjoyable. A ride called One Fish-Two Fish was similar to the Merry -Go-Round except each fish would spray a person with water either from the top fish or the bottom fish as you passed by. The little girl seated next to me enjoyed seeing me get wet. I had fun too. It was a very hot day so it did not take long to dry after the ride. There was an indoor roller coaster and if I knew that in advance I would not have been enticed to participate. Some of those rides the parents enjoyed while I watched the 18 month old child. She did not mind being without her parents as long as I was with her. We went to the other parks that are a part of Disney World also.

The year 2010 began like the weather. In fact in many ways life is like the weather changeable with sunny days, rain, snow, wind, and very stormy days. My body is reacting accordingly.

On January 11th, I entered the hospital with a so-called 'mini stroke'. I got up one morning and the floor felt like I was standing on foam rubber. My mind was confused and I could not get a sense of direction.

On October 21st another trip to the hospital   with a mini heart attack, this time the hospital wanted to send me to a rehabilitation hospital because I had no one at home to care for me. With part time care I went home. On November 4th the cartilage in my knee wore out. This last set back has confined me to home a great deal of time. I try to focus on some type of recovery because I know attitude is important to overcome adversity.

THE GOLDEN YEARS

Youth is beautiful and enjoyable but it does not last forever. Each day brings you closer to the Golden Days (so called) which are difficult. How you manage those years are up to you. Overcoming multiple adversities one at a time gives a person strength through each survival. A good attitude is very important. Many injuries or illnesses cause severe pain. Even after recovery we may find it difficult to do chores that once were possible. In addition to our physical condition we may have to experience humility. I thought about the first time that I was completely uncovered and someone had to wash my body. I pictured Eve (in the Bible story) in the garden of paradise after she ate of the forbidden fruit. She reached for a fig leaf which hardly served the purpose. In today's world the bikini is not that much more of a cover up. However, when you are older this can be very uncomfortable. Today I have come to grips with my health conditions and I am grateful for whatever assistance I receive. Attitude is the thing—it is the way you look at yourself at this point of your life. You may have suffered many losses. The loss of your loved ones may top your list. Your own physical loss of hearing, your eyes not quite as good, difficult to hold objects, to walk very slow and maybe not possible at all. Try to think about what you could do to replace the things you no longer can do. Perhaps a former hobby or an idea that might be helpful to do something in a new way will work wonders.

My generation is very different than the current time. It was a time when people were self-reliant, independent, caring, helpful and respectful of others and their property. There are still good people today that have some of these qualities which are part of my character.

In the chapters of this book I revealed how I survived trauma, grief and my struggles with cancer without a family, no relatives and a few friends. I lived alone and I admit depression took a strong hold on me but basically I was a positive person. I made a decision to find a manner to meet and beat these setbacks. My dad was a great example of courage and will always be an inspiration to me. My goal in writing this book was to leave this world and instrument of Hope and Inspiration. If I accomplished this for you then my efforts have been successful. A New York Yankee baseball player used the phrase, "It is not over until it is over." Attitude is very important to have determination to overcome adversity one at a time. I had dreams of what I wanted to see and do with my life. It would be active and fulfilling. Storms would pass, the sun would shine. It is called HOPE. Nearly everyone has dreams... do not let them die without trying to find a way to accomplish them. Every day is a gift from God... Try to enjoy each day as much as possible.

SOME CLOSING THOUGHTS

What does the spirit of giving mean? To the average person it usually means giving money. This is not necessarily true. The spirit of giving in the form of an encouraging word, a complement, a warm smile, a thoughtful phone call can work wonders in making some one happy. In fact, it would be nice if this practice could continue all year long. This gift of self will mean a great deal to a person living alone and/or surviving a chronic ailment. Those who do volunteer services see the results of such acts. This thoughtful act on your part will reduce the pain of loneliness considerably. You may still be alone but not always lonely. My involvement as a volunteer person has given me many moments of happiness and I have witnessed the effects of such contacts on those I visited. If you would want a volunteer to visit you I would suggest a contact with a church or volunteer group such as Interfaith and there are similar groups. You may even establish a new friendship. The person who lives alone may find himself or herself in this situation either by choice or frequently by circumstance. The emotion of loneliness is felt when a person thinks that he or she is not needed and more often not loved. What can you do if you feel lonely during the holidays or at any time during the year? There are many methods to break the barrier of being alone or lonely. The phone is one of my methods because you can exchange words as if the person were visiting you in your own home. You may not be able to leave your home because of illness. If this is the problem call a church or an organization to provide you with a new contact. Reflect on the real meaning of the holiday instead of looking at the day with its commercial values. I remember my first Christmas Day alone when my last family member died. I went to a restaurant for dinner and sat alone at a table. The place was crowded and filled with laughter. Many thoughts rushed through my mind. Occasionally the waitress came to the table with a friendly smile and exchanged a few words. I went home after the delicious dinner. The quietness when I arrived home was paralyzing. Then as I played some soft music, tears fell. As I recalled my joys of the past, the solitude provided me with consolation. The waitress with the smile that Christmas Day gave me the gift of herself. I frequently go to restaurants, not only for the good food, but also because management, the staff and all the waitresses treat me as if I were part of the family. I would like to acknowledge and to thank all these good people for the many acts of kindness and service given to me.

Many years ago I read an article that I would like to quote. I am grateful to the unknown author and agree with them wholeheartedly.

"The thing that goes the farthest

Towards making life worthwhile

That cost the least and does the most:

Is just a PLEASANT SMILE"

The spirit of giving seems to snowball during the Christmas season. The practice of giving a deserved complement or smile could make someone happy at any time.

IN CONCLUSION

Many people are given a life of relatively good health which is often taken for granted. They seem not to appreciate the joy, love, companionship or the kindness of strangers, who open doors for them or for the disabled persons, until they experience pain, suffering and loneliness. All of these elements are the ingredients of which life is composed. For the present, you could be greatly rewarded by seeing a smile on the face of the person for whom you performed a kindness. Hopefully, the various methods I used to survive my many trials and traumas will prove helpful to you. The main purpose of this book will be fulfilled if only YOU are helped to achieve a better life.

I would like to make a statement here. My dad survived Colon Cancer for twenty years following his cancer surgery. This is remarkable because medical science was not as advanced in the treatment of cancer at that time compared to current times. After surgery Dad resumed his performance of charitable works for his family, friends and even strangers. He enriched the lives of many people by his pleasant manner, thoughtfulness and numerous good deeds. My dad filled his life to the very end serving people. He survived his cancer and died of pneumonia!

There is one new practice which I have established since my Cancer surgery. I have found it very helpful and refreshing to set aside about fifteen minutes each day for myself for QUIET TIME! I sit down, close my eyes and picture some of the beautiful scenes of my past vacations. I visualize lakes with sailboats, fields of pretty tulips or other beautiful flowers. At times I have reflected on my working years when I ate my lunch on a park bench overlooking Lake Michigan. I watched people playing ball on the grass nearby. This even helped me to go back to the office in a little more relaxed state. The time of which I allow myself now to relax gives me new strength. It is so refreshing to escape a fast, noisy World! To some degree, IT IS TAKING THE TIME OUT TO SMELL THE ROSES AND ENJOY LIFE!

My parents taught me from a very young age to appreciate the beauty of the world. Like everyone else, I too, in time got caught up with the tensions of this busy world. However, my family believed in yearly vacations and would enjoy even the simple vacation of going to parks or visiting flower gardens. A Sunday afternoon watching the local baseball game at the park was something we all enjoyed. This is how I learned the game and could understand the plays even by listening to it on the radio. No television just mind visualization.

In later years we had a chance to travel and take longer vacations. The credit for the idea of using those past enjoyable times to relax really belongs to my psychologist, Dr. Gerald Hodan, who taught me the importance of relaxation. Stress caused my cancer. I received literature prior to my radiation treatments to inform me how to build up my immune system. Small changes in my diet would include more fruits, vegetables and whole grains. The book encouraged exercise and recreational activities, music or a hobby to control stress. This was no problem for me because of my involvement with people. I am aware that a positive mental attitude does improve the immune system and thereby helps the body to heal. I have had the return of cancer a few times when I suffered from extreme stress again. I have learned how to defeat stress and rebuild a weakened immune system. ATTITUDE DOES AFFECT HEALTH. There are two ways of looking at life. Look for the bright side – it is not easy. However, it is worth the effort to improve your health – Attitude is the name of the game.

A Book Review From A Friend

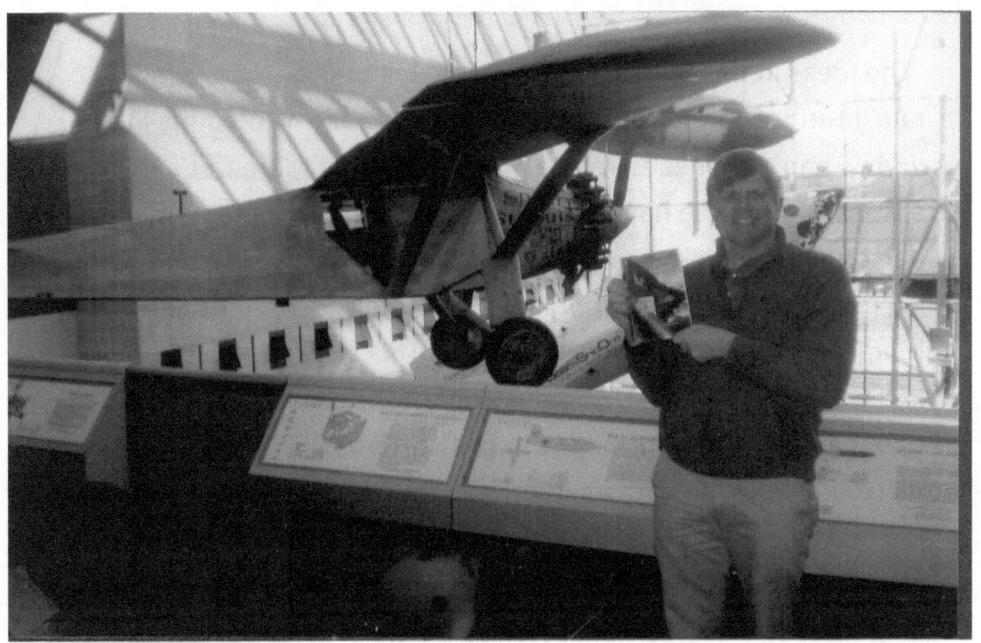

When my very dear friend Steve Kraeger visited the Smithsonian Museum in Washinton, D.C. he took a picture of Charles Linbergh's plane "The Spirit of St. Louis". He thought it would be nice to have this picture appear in my book.   Steve had seen parts of my book before completion and found the contents very interesting and enjoyable.

Professional Reviews

"The ideas in this book have given me will to live. I have faced so much turmoil in the recent months that I really wanted my life to end. I had a chance to read a proof version of Margaret's book and I saw how she handled these situations in her life. I made a personal decision to change my attitude about my situation, imagining how I might find happiness when the rough times pass. If Margaret could do it , why couldn't I? This book is easy to read and ends with a very strong and viable conclusion. Congratulations Margaret on reaching your goals. You have already touched more than one life with your writing, for me the effect has helped me make decisions that have improved my will to live and the courage to take on even greater challenges." - Amy Mueller, Audio/Visual Specialist & Creative Writer.